12 Changes A Year

the recipe book to the

Number Crunch Diet

**When you take control of the numbers
you take control of your weight.**

Volume 1

Jumper Publications and Media

Other Publications

ABC Water and the Number Crunch Diet
a step by step solution to alkaline deficiency and
with a New and Unique approach to weight control

JPM Oral Hygiene Protocol
stop using toxic drugstore mouthwash, discover how to reduce
your gum pocket depth from 3-4-3 to 1-2-1 mm when they probe

NCD Flaxseed Shake Recipe
the Number Crunch Diet method for getting omega 3s
and with three variations so you'll never get bored

Nontoxic Teeth Whitening and Dental Hygiene System
"Spare me the chemicals, I've switched to FOOD GRADE to
whiten, gargle and brush."

The 5 Points of Posture
the missing link to fat loss, overall wellness, and
to becoming Respected, Adored, and Wealthy

12 Changes A Year – Volume 2
the recipe book to the Number Crunch Diet
Begin today and forever be in control of the numbers you're eating.

Vision Is Possible
Improve your vision and get a facelift for free!
an original vision program targeting your Eye Lids

To purchase additional copies, please visit

http://www.CreateSpace.com/4806738

CONTENTS

12 Changes A Year

Volume One

"Reality-Show Recipes"

for the person who wants real cooking

Edits & Format

You will notice oddities in punctuation, spelling, syntax, and perhaps even semantics, within this book. Feel free to let me know, but some of it is done for brevity or to shift emphasis. I use capitals where I see fit, to grab your attention and make it stand out, and I also remove capitals when I don't think they are deserving of them, or to remove emphasis after first usage, i.e., Pyrex becomes pyrex. And french bread, brussels sprouts, and english cucumbers, are spelled lowercase, as we are not going to "link" a European vacation to our food and eating.

Secondly, I will unhyphenate to create rhythm. Grammatically, two or more words that function as an adjective before a noun are supposed to be hyphenated. That's fine. A million-dollar smile, is the adjective "million-dollar" describing the smile. However, this can get redundant after a while, 1&2 3, 1&2 3, 1&2 3. The noun gets all the attention. But what if you want the adjectives to have the emphasis? After all, the adjectives are the descriptive words. So, I will drop the hyphens to allow the adjectives equal emphasis, and to change the pace of the sentence a bit. So if there are no hyphens, read it slower and evenly, one two three four five six seven. A "step-by-step solution" sounds a bit skippy and simplistic, whereas, a "step by step solution" is said slower and sounds more methodical. Hyphenating two words, or joining two words as a compound word, reduces their individual meanings.

With regard to fastfood, healthfood, and seasalt, it's time for these words to evolve into compound words, so the trend starts here.

There are also some fragmented sentences, subject-verb disagreements, and singular/plural violations. When "correcting" certain of these sentences, they lost their emphasis and punch, so I kept them as is.

In the past I've been guilty of judging other author's sentences, only to reread it with the commas, pauses, and then it made perfect sense. So, if there's a comma, then pause, as you may not get to pause later in the sentence. If there's no comma, then don't pause and read it all as one.

I pose questions, but without question marks. Some are rhetorical, but some are to make you Ponder. Great word. Ponder. If you see a question mark at the end, then it requires an answer. If there's no question mark, then you can just say, yeah, no, or hm.

English continues to change, people using it, customize the language to fit what they want to communicate, emphasize, and to make their point from various angles. It also has to have a variety of melodies and rhythms to keep it from being boring. If you find yourself having to reread a sentence, it may be that it's structured that way for that very reason. So take your time. Don't rush. Let the words digest, so that you absorb the material, and hopefully take some of it and make it a part of your life.

Lastly, you will notice that I customized the headers of every page! This is not something Microsoft Word Starter allows you to do. You can only customize three pages, first, even, and odd. So, to get around this I had to create a Page Break every three pages, and as a result, the last line of some of the pages doesn't "justify" to the edge. So I hope that flipping through the upper corners of the pages will assist you in finding the chapter that you are looking for.

You won't see any citations from scientific studies or PubMed, because at JPM we look to a higher source for our reference.

God Bless!

Enjoy the Journey

Email me if you have a question, or if you just want to comment. Your purchase comes with 2-years free support and photos.

Barry Ogston, B.Sc., CLS, MLS(ASCP)

You have to crunch the numbers to see what you're really eating.

CHAPTER 1

NCD FLAXSEED SHAKE™

Hi! Welcome Back!

Hopefully you've read *ABC Water and the Number Crunch Diet.* Assuming this to be the case, let me tell you how Awesome! I think you are, as getting good nutrition and maintaining weight through calorie control are, in my opinion, key answers to good health and longevity.

I wish we had a word in our vocabulary for "looking half your age". If you are 40 and look 20, or you're 60 and look 30-ish, this says it all. These people have health, longevity, energy, and this should really be the desired goal. You don't age. Or you don't age much. Not nearly as much as everyone else. You stand out. You're a freak of nature, defying space and time! I say, Go For It!

This chapter, I believe, is a tool in helping you to achieve this goal. The NCD Flaxseed Shake™ is the most amazing of my inventions. Why? Because flax seeds ground fresh and consumed fresh is the only safe guarantee that you will be consuming those unstable "U" shaped omega-3 fatty acids in their true "U" shaped form.

See, saturated fats, like butter and coconut oil, are relatively stable fats. Coconut oil, since it lacks dairy, can last up to two years at room temperature without spoiling. These saturated fatty acids are straight-line chains. No bends, no twists, no contortions.

In a cell membrane, these saturated straight-line fatty acids provide the cell with rigidity. This is good. But within that rigid ring membrane, we need some flexible points. This is where Omega-3 comes in.

The best way to get omega-3 is by grinding fresh organic flax seeds and consuming them right away, or, in my case, I grind two servings, have one now, and one within 24 hours, keeping the second serving in an airtight container in the refrigerator.

It's similar to an apple spoiling after you cut into it, or strawberries gradually going south in a couple of days. Flax seeds, once ground, need to be consumed right away.

The recipe requires four items.
1. organic flax seeds
2. raw whole milk
3. NCD Secret Protein™
4. blackstrap molasses
This is the NCD Molasses Flaxseed Shake™

There are two other versions. The NCD Maple Flaxseed Shake™, where you will substitute Grade B maple syrup for the molasses, and the NCD Honey Flaxseed Shake™, substituting Raw Unfiltered honey for the molasses.

1. Certified Organic Golden Flax Seeds
I purchase this from Bush Creek Organic Foods, on the web at www.bcof.com, (800) 630-5916. This is the best flaxseed at the best price. The label says, "Grown without chemicals, fungicides, herbicides, or pesticides, and involves no genetically modified organisms, GMOs." Then it says, "In order to get the most benefit from your whole flax seeds, grind them fresh and just before using." See, this company understands that omega-3 fat is unstable and spoils quickly once ground – smart people.

The current cost for 12 one-pound bags is $83.88 plus $16.04 UPS shipping, which averages out to $8.33 per bag, and they are still throwing in a free coffee grinder with the 12-bag purchase. Their website has a lot of information about the health benefits of flax seeds and the quality of their product. I am already a believer in flax, but if you still need convincing, I recommend you read their site. This is definitely a great group of farmers. Thank you Bush Creek!

There is only one ingredient, omega golden flax seeds, certified organic. Plus, this part of the country (North Dakota), is away from freeways and air pollution. Any time you can SEE the air, that's not good for crops.

Nutrition Facts
2T 20g
servings per container ~23 (the "~" sign means approximately)
E = 110 calories per 2 Tablespoons/20 grams
F = 70 calories from fat
total Fat = 8g x9 = 72cal (about the same as F=70)(fat x9=cals)
SF = 1g x9 = 9cal of saturated fat
Omega-3 = 3.8g x9 = 34.2cal
Omega-6 = 1.3g x9 = 11.7cal
Omega-9 = 1.8g x9 = 16.2cal
TF = 0 trans fat=0 per NCD rules
Chol = 0mg cholesterol is not found in plant food
Na = 0mg no sodium
K = 170mg some potassium
CHO = 5g x4 = 20 calories of carbohydrate (carb grams x4=cals)
f = 12g x4 = 48 calories of fiber
s = 0g no sugar
Prot = 4g x4 = 16 calories of protein (prot grams x4=cals)
T = 108 total calories

When we add up our three macros, fat carbs prot, 72 + 20 + 16, we get 108 calories, or T = 108. This is pretty close to the E = 110, but labels aren't perfect. The energy is listed in calories at the top, but you should always calculate it yourself by adding up the fat carbs protein. I call this T, total calories. Also notice the discrepancy in F, fat cals = 70 and our calculated fat cals of 72.

The fiber calories of 48 is higher than the total carb calories of 20, so you may ask, how can this be? I called them and they said that the government makes the Nutrition Facts, they just send the product in for analysis. This leads us to the whole debate about whether you CAN subtract the fiber calories from the carb number. Brace yourselves, as I'll do the best I can.

Insoluble fiber doesn't get absorbed, it stays within the colon, adding bulk to your stool, so it has no calories. Soluble fiber gets absorbed into the body, so it has calories, but it creates a gel gelatin like material that slows down the glycemic load of your meal.

In the USA, the FDA says that companies can subtract the insoluble-fiber grams from the total-carb grams. In Canada, food companies cannot. So, if you buy food in the United States, the manufacturer has likely already subtracted the insoluble fiber from the carbs so you don't want to do it again when you crunch your numbers.

However, there is no consistency and no indication that food companies are doing this and if so which ones are and which ones aren't. This is the gray area of the food label, and so we have to rely on our body's signals and intuition.

If you feel "low energy" after a meal, chances are there weren't enough sugar carbs, or, the soluble gel fiber is slowing down the release of sugar too much. Therefore, you will want to increase the carbs slightly by 3-4% to 43 or 44%. This way, when you subtract the fiber carbs, you end up with closer to 40% carbs.

If the meal leaves you feeling a bit bloated, that "fat gain" feeling, your meal may have too many sugar carbs and the glycemic load is a bit high. In this situation, you will NOT subtract the fiber carbs from your total carbs.

You can also eat the meal slower if you find it has high sugar and it's making you feel fat after eating it. The NCD Shakes have some sugar. Maple syrup, molasses, and honey are powerful sugars. But they are also healthy sugars. This brings us to the:

NCD Five Healthy Sugars™
1. Molasses – blackstrap
2. Maple Syrup – grade B
3. Honey – raw, unfiltered
4. Fruit
5. Cane Sugar – organic, minimally refined

Molasses is unrefined syrup from sugarcane or sugar beets.
Grade B maple syrup, tree sap, is less refined than grade A.
Honey, raw unfiltered, is unrefined sugar from a beehive.
Fruit, fresh in-season fruit is packed with nutrients and color.
Cane sugar is partially refined, but needed in certain recipes.

I tried agave cactus syrup, but it seemed a bit refined, and brown rice syrup, same thing. So I narrowed it down to this list of five. These are the most unrefined, mineral rich, nutrient dense. And cane sugar is needed in certain recipes just because molasses, maple syrup, honey, and fruit, don't work. Blackstrap molasses, dark maple syrup, and raw honey, spell minerals, minerals, and nutrients, plus fruit, and the cane sugar. These NCD Five Healthy Sugars™ are all you need for sweetener. And some organic stevia occasionally.

So back to our fiber. Do we subtract or do we not subtract? With the NCD we crunch the numbers both ways so we can see the meal and the percent macros with the fiber included and with the fiber subtracted. Then the rest is intuition. If the meal has fiber and not enough sugar, you'll be back at the refrigerator shortly after you've eaten. A 35-30% carb meal will make you lose fat a bit faster, but you may feel low energy. A 50-60% carb meal may make you feel like you need to get on the treadmill and burn off some calories. We will crunch the recipes both ways, regular and subtracted, and then look at the whole meal for a best estimate that targets 40% carbs. There's just no way to know EXACTLY whether you can subtract the fiber calories or not. But this is good, because it's making you pay more attention to your body signs. Your Internals.

CHAPTER 2

NCD Omega 3 Protocol™

You will take one 454g 16oz bag of Bush Creek flax seeds and aliquot it, (divide it up), into ten 2oz SKS glass jars with the screw caps, 46g each. If you didn't buy the SKS glass jars mentioned in the *ABC Water and the Number Crunch Diet*, you can grind 23g directly from the bag each time you prepare a shake, or you can grind 46g from the bag, and use 23g and store the remaining 23g in some sort of airtight container that you have. The one-pound bag contains about 460g of flax seeds, so, 10x46g=460g. They give you a few extra grams. It is important to verify the weight of the food products you will be using. The six-pack of french-bread rolls says one roll is 71 grams, but they consistently make them 85-91g, so you are getting 46 more carb calories than you might think. I was tricked by this "one roll 71g" on the label, until I checked it.

The flaxseed bag is opaque, so no light gets in, and it has a ziplock so you can reseal it. Store them in the refrigerator. The website says the seeds will last indefinitely if stored sealed, protected from light, in the refrigerator, unground. If you have one Flaxseed Shake per day, then you will finish the bag in 20 days, 1/20th of the bag per shake. If you have 20 flaxseed shakes a month, then after one year you will have eaten 12 pounds of flax seeds! This is some serious omega-3 therapy. And of the highest quality, and consumed the most beneficial way, FRESHLY GROUND.

Contrast this with the vast majority of the population who aren't eating flax seeds at all, or properly. This, and all of your other JPM strategies will have you looking HYA – HALF YOUR AGE!!

Ok, so we aliquoted our bag of flax seeds into 10 x 46g, and each aliquot of 46g will yield 2 servings of 23g for a total of 20 shakes.

Now, our Nutrition Facts label was for 20g, but for our shake we will be using 23g. This is 3g more. Don't get scared, just watch how I do this.

$23/20 = 1.15$

We are going to multiply all our Nutrition Facts numbers by 1.15.

23g
E=110x1.15=126.5=127 calories
F=70x1.15=80.5=81 calories
total Fat=72x1.15=82.8=83 calories
SF=9x1.15=10.4=10 calories
Omega-3 = 34.2x1.15=39 calories
Omega-6 = 11.7x1.15=13 calories
Omega-9 = 16.2x1.15=19 calories
TF=0
Chol=0
Na=0
K=170x1.15=196mg
CHO=20x1.15=23 calories
f=48x1.15=55 calories
s=0
Prot=16x1.15=18 calories
T= 83+23+18 = 124 calories

Are you okay? Some people are terrified of math. It's okay. It's just new at first, and then it's mindless repetition. Remember, you'll be miles ahead of the average person after a while when it comes to number crunching. Chances are, it will spill over into other areas, like, for example, you may stop forgetting where you put your car keys.

We will do this again, so no worries. But when you divide up a package of food, you have to recalculate the nutrition facts to match your new serving size. That's all we did.

Notice that the Nutrition Facts label gives you the fat in calories, F, but then it also gives you the fat in grams, Total Fat. This is another place where you will see a little discrepancy. In the above, the F = 81 but the total F = 83.

The new Nutrition Facts label will no longer have the F, (fat in calories), listed. So if you want to know the number of calories of fat, you will have to take the Total Fat in grams and multiply it by 9. Removing the Fat Cals is a bad move. If I pick up meat lasagna and the calories are 420 and the fat cals are 210, that tells me easily and quickly that the product is 50% fat, it goes back on the shelf.

When it comes to calculating the T, Total Calories at the bottom, I will use the total Fat in grams x9 number. So, 83+23+18=124 calories. The E at the top was 127. As you get comfortable with the label you will see how you can double-check their numbers and see discrepancies. Most of the time it's just slight.

Now let's go deeper with the numbers. Recall our example from the *ABC Water and the Number Crunch Diet*, Chapter 57, "Crunch Time!" If I have $1.00 total and I have 4 dimes, what percent of my money is dimes? 0.40/1.00=0.40x100=40%

If I have 83 fat calories, and 124 total calories, what's the percent fat? 83/124x100=67%

If I have 23 carb calories and 124 T calories, what's the percent carbs? 23/124x100=18.5% or 19% rounded off.

If I have 18 prot cals and 124 T cals, what's the percent protein? 18/124x100=15%

The marcos are 19 67 15. It should add up to 100 or 100%, but we rounded up twice, so 19+67+15=101. No biggie. If your three macro percents add up to 102, you made a calculation error, recrunch.

So flax seeds are 67% fat or about 2/3rds fat, as we would expect from seeds. They have some protein 15% and some carbs 19%.

Now most labels won't have a breakdown of omega 3 6 9, but this is an omega food, high in omega-3, so they have the three plant fats listed.

Our 23g serving of flaxseed has 39 calories of omega-3. What's the percent? 39/124x100=31%

FLAX SEEDS ARE 31% OMEGA 3 !!!!!!!!!!!!!!!!

Flax Seeds are almost 1/3rd Omega 3 !!!!!!!!!!!!!!!!!

Now are you getting it? Do you see how this is so critical to your diet? This is THEE way to get fresh stable U-shaped omega-3 fat.

DHA and EPA from cod liver oil, and Omega-3 from Flax Seeds.

Chia seeds are #2 and Hemp seeds are #3 for omega-3 content. I've never tried chia seeds, but they are imported from Mexico, South America, and Australia, and I would rather support my North and South Dakota organic flaxseed farmers. On page 53, Udo Erasmus, the PhD fat expert, states in *Fats That Heal Fats That Kill*, that hemp seeds contain only trace amounts of THC, tetrahydrocannabinol, cannabis, marijuana, but it is possible that it could show up in a urine drug screen. None-the-less, hemp seeds are loaded with minerals, good fat, and nearly 25% protein. You will enjoy an 8oz bag of raw organic hemp seeds with the NCD Orange Chicken™ recipe.

Your next sources of omega-3 are nuts, walnuts being the highest, but nowhere near the amount found in flax seeds. So, flax seeds win. And the NCD Flaxseed Shake™ is the ideal way to consume them.

The omega-6 percent in a 23g serving is 13/124x100=10%.
The omega-9 percent in a 23g serving is 19/124x100=15%.

Now what if we wanted to convert our 39 calories of omega-3 into grams? What would we do? Well, we used x9 to go from grams to calories, so it's divide by 9 to go back. 39/9=4.3g omega-3.

So each shake has 4.3g of omega-3 fat. This would be like 4.3 very large fish oil or salmon oil capsules, 1000mg each. Now, fish oil and flax are not the same, but this is just to give you an idea of how much 4.3 grams of omega-3 fat is. If you were taking 1000mg flax oil capsules, then one shake would have 4.3 capsules. Most people can't stomach all those capsules. Plus the oil is refined from the seeds, so you are losing nutrition, and gaining contaminants and rancidity.

The NCD says, eat as close to the original food as possible. In this case, eat the actual seeds, ground fresh.

I tried flaxseed oil, I didn't like it. And it spoiled quickly. That's the key trait of omega-3 fat, and fish oil. They're unstable fats.

So you have all the advice givers saying "eat more omega-3s" and never giving you exactly how to do it. Here it is.

JPM – from Advice to Results™

The advice givers also repeatedly say "Healthy Fats". If you've read *ABC Water and the Number Crunch Diet*, you know inside and out, the difference in fats and what a healthy and unhealthy fat is. It says right on the front of the book "new dietary fat categories". Read the book. It's a compilation of nearly 100 books that I've read in the past 13 years, each author having their own specialized area of health knowledge, and I've synergized that knowledge into a completely new area – Selfcare Protocols.

Lastly, our saturated fat is 10 calories per 23g serving shake. What is the percent? 10/124x100=8%

So, as you can see, the fat in flax seeds is 31% omega-3, 10% omega-6, 15% omega-9, and 10% saturated.   God made this food for a specific purpose in MIND.   Omega-3

Chapter Endnote
Coming up, you are going to see "less-than" and "greater-than". Initially, I spelled them as two separate words, but when I saw Wikipedia spelling them with hyphens, it occurred to me that, yes, we say it as a unit, and it sounds better as "lessthan" rather than "less than".   Grammarians will disagree, oh well.

Also, you may have noticed that when there's a quotation within a sentence, that I place the comma on the outside of the quotation mark.   Many writers and grammarians say you should place the comma inside the quotation.   However, this gives the impression that the comma is part of the quotation.   I keep my quotations "clean", and place the comma on the outside.   Sorry grammarians.

Lastly, the word "thee" means you.   Unfortunately, dictionaries don't have a word for "thē", the with a long e.   When you say "the" with a long e, people understand this to mean "exclusively". Perhaps one day, dictionaries will update their definition of "thee" to say, 16th century "you", modern day "exclusively", or "only".

Page 264, *ABC Water and the Number Crunch Diet*
EPA = Eicosapentaenoic = i-co-sa-penta-en-no-ic Acid
DHA = Docosahexaenoic = doe-co-sa-hexa-en-no-ic Acid

Use those words in a sentence at your next employee potluck and you'll gain a whole new look of respect.

And then when they ask you why you don't refer to them as Omega-3s.   Tell them, flax, chia, and hemp seeds have three double bonds whereas EPA and DHA have 5 and 6 double bonds.   They're not the same molecules, and although they have overlapping roles, they also have uniquely different functions.

CHAPTER 3

Milk & Ellen White

I like to keep the chapters on the short side so that you stop and let it sink in. It's when you stop to ponder, that's when your mind starts planning how it can add this into your lifestyle.

Now recall that omega-3 can convert to DHA and EPA fish oil, our good hormones. The rate is small, 2.7%, but better than nothing. So our flaxseed shake with its 39 calories 4.3 grams of omega-3 can make about 116mg of EPA. This would be about 1/5th of a teaspoon of cod liver oil. Not very much, but at least it's something. This is why we need both, flax and fish oil. Flax for membranes and fish oil for hormones. At one time they referred to flax seeds as "vegetarian fish oil", but it doesn't convert enough.

On the other hand, this is still uncharted territory, and there may be people who can convert flax omega-3 into fish oil DHA EPA at 10-20-30%. The great news is that omega-3 can convert to fish oil.

This again is why we do not call fish oil omega-3. Nor do we use the words "mono" and "polyunsaturated". Chapter 49 ABC NCD, dietary fats defined.

NCD Edible Fats™
3 6 9 plants
saturated animal fat and coconut oil
fish fat

Come on America! And the rest of the world! Get on board!
Imagine what could happen if people stopped consuming fryer oil?

2. Raw Milk
I buy mine at Lassen's Health Foods and from Organic Pastures
Dairy in Fresno, California. Thank you to both of these great
companies for fighting to keep raw milk on the shelves. In fact,
more people are buying it than ever before. This milk is so
beneficial. Read their website at www.organicpastures.com, it's
very very impressive. The founder/owner invented a mobile
milking machine so he can milk the cows out in the pasture and not
in a barn. I am sure you've seen pictures of some dairies. You
can't label all milk as bad. People that do that are just dumb. Raw
milk is good food – "Time Test" passed.

The label says, "We don't pasteurize or homogenize this perfect
raw food." It also boasts that it's a natural source of good bacteria
probiotics, so by drinking this milk I have no need for probiotic
supplementation. Good gut flora is essential to good health. Raw
milk provides this. It's USDA certified organic, meaning, no
hormones, no antibiotics in the feed, no sewer sludge used to grow
the feed, et cetera. That "sewer sludge" that Los Angeles ships up
here for nonorganic farming is about as good a reason as any to buy
organic. And if the spray pesticides and GMOs weren't bad
enough, now they want to irradiate the food to extend the shelf life.

I hope you can see the difference in the two types of food available
for you to eat. Normal traditional food made in line with nature
and God, and the other being man's way, adulterated, and seems to
be getting freakier with every passing few years. I bought some
eggnog a few years ago and the word "Cloned" was on the carton.
It read, "Not from cloned dairy." And it wasn't a joke. It was a
serious statement on the container. God help us if that's where
we're heading.

The raw milk from Organic Pastures does come in a plastic jug, but
this conscientious company has informed its customers that "Our
plastic bottles are free of BPA, bisphenol A, and no phthalates,

13

plasticizers." This is such a great company. All dairy producers should model themselves after this company. Berkeley Farms is another brand I buy sometimes, if I buy regular milk. It tastes good and I don't ever have a reaction. The company was established in 1910, so I like that it's been around for more than a century, and it says "Passionate about Purity" on the label. There's that "Purity" thing again. Even the milk producers are chiming in on it. Why? Because HEAVY METAL CONTAMINATION, or any and all sorts of contamination and pollutants and things that shouldn't be in your food and supplements are getting in. Pay attention to Purity. That's my advice. And know who you are buying from. And know the history of the companies you buy from.

"Oh, it's vegetable oil spread now, it's okay, it's not like the old margarine." Oh really.

And soft drink machines selling a 20oz cola for $1.00 that cost maybe 5 cents to make, what do you think of a company like this?

Vote with your dollars. Vote out the bad and vote in the good.

Raw milk also provides raw proteins, unheated, undenatured. The NCD is big on raw, aim for 80% raw and 20% cooked, and only cooked to MW (medium-well) or 3/4ths done, then allow it to finish cooking off heat to just right. We don't want rogue misshapened denatured proteins activating our immune system.

I can tolerate most brands of regular milk, (pasteurized homogenized), but there is one brand that consistently gives me bad GI reactions. This is dirty dairy milk. Cow butt bacteria is getting into the milk. Yuck. Bad Bacteria. I won't tell you the brand, but just be aware that there are many different kinds of cow's milk. Find a good one and start drinking it.

You will need a half gallon, 64oz, of whole milk for the recipe.
Nutrition Facts
1cup 240mL
servings per container 8

E=150cal
F=70cal
total Fat=8g x9=72cal   47%
SF=5g x9=45cal
TF=0
Chol=30mg
Na=105mg
CHO=12g x4=48cal   32%
f=0
s=12g x4=48cal
Prot=8g x4=32cal   21%
T=152

Okay, so 72+48+32=152 calories total. Our E at the top is 150, so it's close. F=70 and we calculated 72. Notice I placed the percent macros out to the right a bit, 47% fat 32% carbs 21% protein.

Try crunching them.   72/152x100=47% fat, 48/152x100=32% carbs, 32/152x100=21% protein.

0.5 rounds up, and 0.49 rounds down. Standard math rule.

Recall that our NCD Emergency Meal™ is 2% milk, 16oz is a snack, 250 calories, and one quart would be a meal, ~500 calories.

Whole milk is of course more milk fat. It's 32 47 21. Higher in milk fat and lower in protein and lower in carbs. This is a weight-gain food because the 32% carbs is all sugar. That sugar raises insulin and the whole thing gets converted into body fat.

Our 2% milk is more macro balanced. It was very close to the target 40 30 30, it was 38 33 29, see page 274 of the ABC NCD.

The higher protein, 29%, and lower fat, 33%, makes this less of a weight gainer. Although, you can still gain weight from 2% milk because all the carbs are sugar carbs. So you just drink it slower. Take it to your desk and drink it over an hour, a one-hour infusion. Then it becomes a nice long healthy satisfying meal. With an added benefit of minerals and hydration. A cow's sole purpose on this planet is to chew green grass all day long to make milk for humans. Chickens make eggs. How can you deny these foods?

I am going to speak to the Seventh-Day Adventists for a moment. Now I am a big believer in SDA principles and teachings. I even installed my own Glory Star satellite dish. For $200 you get FREE television for the rest of your life. Pay for the dish and pay nothing after that, no monthly charge, Great Deal! Glory Star satellite TV programming by the Three Angels Network, www.3ABN.org.

Toss your current TV provider in the trash, pay no monthly fees, and get better quality television. They will teach you about real history, real news, and, well, the real God. I'm not apologizing for that one.

So my Beef with SDA is this. Here's where they got it wrong about vegetarianism. Ellen White, the author and teacher of SDA principles, was ill. So she switched to an all fruit-and-vegetable diet and got well. Here's where today's SDAs get it wrong.

The all fruit-and-vegetable diet is for when you are ill.™

If you are not ill, you should be eating plants and animals.™

A healthy person can eat and tolerate all kinds of foods. It's also referred to as a "steel gut". A weak person can't eat this and can't eat that. That's not a healthy person.

Ellen White promoted veganism because she was ill and it made her well. Basically, she balanced her acid-base balance. She stocked up her alkaline reserves. She could have done the same thing by drinking the ABC Water for a source of bicarbonate base.

Seventh-Day Adventists misinterpret this to mean, that healthy people should eat a vegan diet. No. Sick people should eat a vegan diet. It's an alkaline diet, and most sickness symptoms are rooted in what? What? What is the root of most sickness and disease? Low alkalinity and high acidity in the body.

ALKALINE DEFICIENCY™
If you've read ABC NCD then you get this. Yay! You get it!

But not just "yay you get it", but "yay you get THE REASON WHY YOU DON'T FEEL WELL AND YOU'RE AGING."

ALKALINE DEFICIENCY ALKALINE DEFICIENCY ALKALINE DEFICIENCY

Never mind alkaline foods, just eat according to the NCD and track your urine pH to see where you're at – Chapter 10 ABC NCD.

So my fellow SDAs, you misinterpreted Ellen White's situation. The vegetarian diet is the "Get Well" diet. If you are well and healthy, then your next goal should be to become fit; strong flexible muscles with a great cardiovascular system, a gymnast, a diver, speed skater, hurdler. That's going to take some protein, 30%. Beans are 40% protein, but lean chicken, tuna, fish, turkey, and ham are 90-100% protein, lean pork chops are 75% protein, and lean beef is 2/3rds protein.

So there you have it. I just debunked the foundational dietary principle of the Seventh-Day Adventist religion. Ellen White used it because she was sick and it made her well. It's a Get-Well diet.

Ellen could have likely gotten better by supplementing with bicarbonate to fix her acidosis. But she likely needed the phytonutrients and the natural plant minerals and vitamins as well.

The two go hand in hand. God made both plants and animals. And we've been eating both for as long as time is recorded. Jesus ate fish with his bread, and I'll bet he drank cow's or goat's milk when he needed a quick snack.

We are going to use 1 cup 240mL 8oz of whole milk per flaxseed shake. So half a gallon will make eight shakes.

3. Fat Free Cottage Cheese

Sadly, the Trader Joe's brand now has "Natural Flavor". Shame Shame. So to get cottage cheese without Titanium Dioxide and Natural Flavor, you have to buy organic. Organic cottage cheese is now in the same price category as meat, fish, and poultry. And I have noticed that foods with protein cost more. It's like "someone" is making protein expensive for the average person. It's like "someone" is trying to get the average everyday person to eat inexpensive grains and junk foods. Does cottage cheese really need to be made with so much crap? Mono and diglycerides, locust bean gum, guar gum, xanthan gum, carrageenan, titanium dioxide, artificial flavor, natural flavor. And you will never convince me that "Natural Flavor" is raspberry flavoring extracted from fresh berries. Give me a break. The NCD says it's "Chemicals That Make You, and Me, Addicted To The Food Product." If it weren't for some of these "Exposers" we'd never know half the stuff that's going on in our world.

So plan on budgeting more for food in the future, as unadulterated food is going to be for the wealthy and the elite. Middle-class food for the middle class, and poor food for the poor. The New Normal.

Next Chapter Note

Throughout all JPM books, chemical compounds are hyphenated, just be aware that the standard rule is to spell them as separate words. If you say them together, with the hyphen, the sentence should flow better. Hopefully!

Also, there are two camps when it comes to hyphenating fractions. One group says, do not hyphenate if the denominator functions as a noun, only hyphenate if the fraction functions as an adjective. The other group says you should hyphenate all fractions regardless. I decided to go with the second camp, since, as a number, it's 2 slash 3, then as a written word it makes more sense to be two hyphen three. Also, as a noun, "two" is not modifying "thirds", the fraction is a unit, "two-thirds". While we're on the subject of math, if you see "~", read the word "about" or "approximately", ~10, about ten.

CHAPTER 4

NCD Mineral Shake™

Yes, this is likely to be the world's record for the longest recipe, more than 20 pages and 4 chapters. Hey, I did say that the NCD would have you looking at the foods you are eating with greater insight. That means detail.

For our 8-shake recipe we will need 4 lbs of nonfat cottage cheese, either 4x1 lb containers or 2x2 lb containers. (454g x4 or 907g x2)

The Nutrition Facts are for ½ a cup 113.5 grams.
I am going to multiply it by 2, so,
1cup 227g
E=160
F=0
total Fat=0   0%
SF=0
TF=0
Chol=0
Na=780mg cottage cheese contains a significant amount of salt
CHO=8g x4=32cal   22%
f=0
s=8g x4=32cal
Prot=28g x4=112cal 78%
T=144cal

So our NFCC is 78% protein. A good way to get protein. It's also a pretty high source of salt. Probably not the good kind, unrefined with natural minerals intact, but rather the white refined tablesalt, or the sodium-phosphate salt. The organic TJs brand has just as much salt. The NCD aims for Na to be <1g per meal. Keeping in mind that salt added is not the same as salt found naturally in the food. The one cup of raw milk has 105mg of naturally-occurring salt, not salt added during manufacturing.

If I have five meals a day, then my maximum salt intake would be 5 grams, naturally occurring and unnaturally added. If the meal has 1300mg of salt, Na=1300, then I do notice a slight thirst sensation after eating it. You would be hard-pressed to find a restaurant meal with less-than 1000mg or 1g of salt. This is why the waitress brings water to the table. You're going to need it later after you finish eating. Foods that contain salt naturally, don't make me thirsty. It's the added salts that make a person thirsty. Again, one word, salt, but lots of different varieties.

Some NCD meals have very little salt, so, by the end of the day, my intake for Na is less-than 3000mg 3g, which is the allowable recommended limit for a 2500-calorie a day diet. And then if you subtract the natural-occurring salt from that 3000mg then my daily "added salt" or "bad salt" is closer to 1500-2000mg, or less.

Chicken breast with the 15% solution is pumped full of sodium-phosphate salt. This and all the other "bad salts" are what raises blood pressure. MSG, monosodium glutamate, sodium phosphate, sodium pyrophosphate, sodium diacetate, you might as well just take a gun and blow your brains out because that is what these sodium salts are doing to the neurons in your head. Sorry, that was a bit strong. But my publisher suggested adding violence to sell more books. Read up on Excitotoxins and you'll see what I mean.

4. And our last ingredient, Molasses.
But as I have discovered, not just any molasses. It has to be Blackstrap and ideally Plantation brand. At the bottom of the Nutrition Facts label lists a few minerals, and what I discovered is, the well-known Grandma's brand that I purchased, because it was

cheaper, lacks minerals. The label says that a 1T serving has 2% of the RDA of calcium and 2% of the RDA of iron. You would think that molasses being unrefined sugar would contain more than that. Well, it does. But not this brand. I then bought the Plantation brand at the healthfood store and a 1T serving has 20% the RDA of calcium and 20% the RDA of iron. That's ten-times more calcium and iron than the regular grocery-store brand. This is why the healthfood store is so much better. It's the details. The devil is in the details, and the devil somehow removed 90% of the minerals. If calcium and iron are ten-times higher in the Plantation brand then you can assume all the other minerals are also ten-times higher. Conversely, if Grandma's brand has 90% less, 2% instead of 20% calcium and iron, then you can assume it has 90% less of all minerals. Maybe it's the soil, or perhaps it's the refining. The organic blackstrap molasses had 10% the RDA for calcium and 15% the RDA for iron and 8% the RDA for magnesium.

Whatever the reason for the difference in mineral content, I suggest you look for one with high minerals, 10-15-20% and not 2%, as the reason we are using this product is for sweetener and for the minerals.

I chose the nonorganic Plantation brand blackstrap unsulphured molasses, 15 fl oz, 442 mL, that came in a glass bottle for $8.49. This is four times as much money as the one in the one-gallon jug at Smart & Final, but without the minerals, you're just getting sugar. So now you know.

You will be pouring 360g of this molasses into your Ninja Blender, divided by 8 servings = 45g of molasses per shake.
E=90
F=0
total Fat=0   0%
SF=0
TF=0
Chol=0
Na=21
K=1286mg this is a high potassium mineral food, good

CHO=94cal   100%
f=0
s=94cal
Prot=0   0%
T=94cal
429mg Calcium
7.7mg Iron

The Nutrition Facts label is for 1T tablespoon 21g.
E=42
Na=10
K=600
CHO=11g
s=11g
Calcium 20% of RDA
Iron 20% of RDA

The RDA for calcium is 1000mg, so 20% is 200mg. There is 200mg of calcium in 1T 21g of this blackstrap molasses. Nice.

The RDA for iron is 18mg, so 20% of 18 is 18x0.20=3.6. There is 3.6mg of iron in 1T 21g of this blackstrap molasses. Good.

Since our recipe uses 45g per serving, I divided 45/21=2.14, and multiplied all the numbers on the nutrition facts by 2.14.

So E=42x2.14=90cal, Na=10x2.14=21mg, K=600x2.14=1286 etc.

By using this brand of molasses, our shake has 429mg of calcium and 7.7mg of iron. Almost half your RDA for both of these minerals. There's your nutrition. That your body needs.

Here's your clue. If you see lots of potassium, then you can assume there are lots of the other minerals as well. My Grandma's brand molasses had 110mg of potassium per 1T, and my Plantation brand has 600mg of potassium per 1T.

Wouldn't it be great if we could have mineral data on the food label so we could see what kind of soil it was grown on and how much refining was done in the making of the food product?

Take some time to review the number crunching we just did. How if your label serving size says 1T 21g and you will be using 45g per Flaxseed Shake, how you have to do 45/21=2.14 and multiply all the numbers on your food label by 2.14, and in the case of the flax seeds we used 23g instead of 20g and did 23/20=1.15 and multiplied the entire label by 1.15. Get comfortable with that.

So our three molasses products are:
A. Grandma's brand – not blackstrap
B. Organic blackstrap
C. Plantation brand – blackstrap, not organic

Notice that I chose the nonorganic brand. For three reasons.
1. it had the highest calcium and iron percents
2. it came in glass
3. it had the lowest carbs

	Container	Calcium	Iron	Carbs
A.	plastic	2%	2%	16g
B.	plastic	10%	15%	14g
C.	glass	20%	20%	11g

Do you see the superior molasses brand?

The Plantation brand came in glass, it had the highest percent calcium and the highest percent iron, and the lowest carbs, 11g.

This is a good company. Vote for them.

The organic molasses came in plastic, it had higher carbs, therefore more refined, sweeter, less robust, and therefore along with more refined comes less minerals, 10% calcium and 15% iron.

The regular-supermarket everyday common brand was higher still in carbs, 16g, with a lot less calcium and iron, more refined.

This took me half a day to analyze, but it means a whole lot to your Divine Intelligence that needs these nutrients to make your body work properly.

If you've read the ABC NCD then you are reading labels. Good. Now the next step is to study and analyze them. This is your master's degree in number crunchology.

The 1 cup of milk in the flaxseed shake has 300mg of calcium, and the 1 cup of NFCC has 200mg of calcium, for a total of 500mg. The 23g of flaxseed has 69mg of calcium, so that's 569mg. Now add to this the 429mg of calcium in the molasses, and you get 998mg of calcium. This shake has ~1000mg of calcium, your recommended daily allowance (well it's RDV now, recommended daily value).

Now if this shake is packed with your RDA of calcium then it's likely to be packed with your RDA for magnesium, zinc, copper, chromium, and all of your other minerals as well. It could just as easily be called the NCD Mineral Shake™. This may be the longest recipe in history, but for a reason. It's packed with nutrition. And we've nearly forgotten about the reason for this shake in the first place, the omega three content! Plus it has 30% protein. This recipe is a masterpiece! Plus it tastes good.

All those people who put kale in their shakes, YUCK. Don't put greens in a shake, because no amount of sugar will make it taste good. They make these shakes on TV and the people take one sip of it and leave the rest. They don't even drink their own shakes! Eat your greens first thing when you get up and get them out of the way, and eat them alone, the NCD Leafy Greens Protocol™, page 250 ABC NCD.

Blending greens into a shake is just about the dumbest thing I've seen people do. You're just asking for Gross.

The NCD Shake Mistake!™

CHAPTER 5

NCD Secret Ingredient™

Time to make a batch of 8 shakes. Are you ready! Grab your Ninja! I hope you bought or already own one. I have the Pro System 1100. It has 6 blades, 2 at the bottom, 2 in the middle, and 2 at the top. You will need all these blades plus the 1100 watts of power to convert the cottage cheese into liquid protein.

NCD Secret Ingredient™
LIQUEFIED Nonfat Cottage Cheese™

This is worth the price of this book, in my opinion.

Have you noticed there's no protein powder in this shake, or any of my recipes? I don't own protein powder. Now I am not against it, but SOOOOO many diet books use protein powder to raise the protein content of their shakes. I came up with a natural way.

Take nonfat cottage cheese and blend it in your Ninja, and voila! You have liquid casein and whey protein – From Food.™

I've never seen or read or heard of anyone doing this, JPM – *Your First Choice for Selfcare Strategies.*

Nonfat cottage cheese is 78% protein. The rest is 22% lactose milk sugar. This 78% protein content is better than a lot of protein powders on the market, some of which are only 40-50% protein or less.   A friend of mine had one and it was so sweet.   When I crunched the numbers, it was 81% carbs sugar, 12% protein, and 7% fat.   Can you say "Protein Powder Scam"?   You get more protein in a peanut-butter sandwich.

You have to crunch the numbers to see what you are really eating, and paying for.™

So none of the NCD recipes, NONE, have protein powder in them. And yet they all contain 30% protein.   I know, it's amazing.

Although I am not against using protein powder, (like the one I referred to on page 93 of the main book), it is a refined product from milk, and it is dry, dehydrated, and a bit lifeless.   If I do start to use it, it will only be a small 25-calorie serving added to about 4oz of raw milk, taken before bed to supply my body with amino acids for muscle synthesis while I sleep.   Not as the protein portion of a meal or shake.

So, place the blade into your Ninja pitcher and then add your two quarts of NFCC.   Place it on the scale and press "on", it will read zero.   Add 360g of your crude blackstrap molasses.   Secure the lid and blend on #2 for 5 minutes.   Set a timer.   The Ninja has three settings, low, medium, and high.   Since we are blending for 5 minutes, I use the medium speed to protect the motor.   It's smooth looking within 2-3 minutes, but I like my liquid cottage cheese to be super smooth, completely blended.

While the timer is ticking, get 8 of your 32oz SKS glass jars with the screw caps.   See page 24 of the main book for where to purchase them.

Now, you will want to record the weight of your empty Ninja pitcher with blade and lid.   Mine's 1137 grams.   So when my five minutes are up, I stop the blender, remove the pitcher from the base and place it on the scale.   Using your calculator, subtract 1137g from the weight, and this is the weight of the pitcher's contents. For me it's about 3329g – 1137g = 2192g divided by 8 = 274g.   So each of my servings is going to be 274g. See how I did that? The blender contains the whole batch of 8 servings, and the contents weighs 2192g, so 2192g/8=274g. So now remove the blender lid, place one of your 32oz jars on the scale, press "tare" to zero it, and pour 274 grams into the jar. Repeat 6 more times. So you now have 7 jars filled and the remaining amount in the blender pitcher is your 8th serving. Pour out as much as you can into the 8th jar. Now place the pitcher on the scale and add 240g of the whole milk. Place the pitcher lid on tight and shake it up-and-down to dissolve the NFCC from the walls of the pitcher. Pour it into your 8th jar. Cap it. Add 240g of the whole milk to each of the remaining 7 jars and cap them. Refrigerate them all. You now have 8 jars of molasses shake. Clean up.

Each of these 8 jars has 1 cup of whole raw milk, 1 cup of NFCC, and 45g of blackstrap molasses.

Time to make a Flaxseed Shake.

Take your 2oz SKS jar with the 46g of flax seeds that we aliquoted earlier. Add the entire 46g to your coffee grinder and grind it for 10-15 seconds, shaking the coffee grinder up-and-down a bit to prevent the flax from sticking to the sides. If you grind longer than 15 seconds your flax seeds will begin to stick to the insides, creating a slight paste. So 10-15 seconds of grinding only. This also mixes the seed so that there are no unground seeds when you are done. Just grinding on the table doesn't mix the seeds enough. So just hold the grinder in your hands and gently shake it as you grind and count to 10. That's it. Stop. Your 46g of flax seeds should be perfectly ground with no sticking to the interior. It will turn into seed butter if you keep grinding it.

While holding the grinder and cap, turn the grinder upside down, tap the side of the grinder with the heel of your hand to dislodge the flax, then slide the grinder out from the cap. You now have 46 grams of ground flaxseed in your cap, cup. Ingenious, I know.

Place the 2oz SKS jar on the scale, zero it, then spoon in 23g of the ground flaxseed. Cap and refrigerate it. This is your second aliquot/serving for later.

The remaining ground flax in your cap cup, is your 23g serving for your shake right now. Add it to the jar of NFCC-milk-molasses. Cap & Shake. Shake it hard with both hands for about 20 seconds. This is your ab workout for the day. Seriously. If you hold your core tight, and shake that jar for 30-45 seconds, you will be out of breath and have sore, tight, rock-hard abs the next day. Do it!

There's a dumbbell called the "Shake Weight". I have two of them. Don't laugh. They work. You won't get huge muscles, but you will definitely wake them up and make them tight. So hold your core tight and shake that jar of your flaxseed shake as hard and as fast as you can for as long as you can. Then open the lid and reward yourself with a drink. Mmm!

Alternatively, you can replace the lid with the "lid with hole" and use your glass drinking straw, page 26 ABC NCD. When you are finished, add a little water to the jar and gently swirl it to wash off the insides so you don't waste any of this nutrition-packed meal.

It's 500 calories and 40% carbs 30% fat 30% protein.

You know, a word of caution about those protein-powder shake formulas. I know a guy who won second place in a weight-loss contest and received a $5000 home gym. A year later he blew up like a balloon, gaining it all back and then some. He said he stopped drinking the protein-powder shakes because it was costing him $100+ a month. Do you see the connection? Cheating never gets you anywhere but back where you started, or worse. Sadly, these companies never tell you what happens when you stop drinking their weight-loss shakes. So now he's in worse shape than before with no knowledge or understanding to get him going in the right direction. It was short lived glory. And a waste of a year.

Four Ingredients

1. NFCC – for lean protein
2. Unrefined sugar – for minerals and sweetness
3. Raw Milk – for protein, fat, carbs, minerals, and PROBIOTICS!
4. Flax Seeds – for omega-3 fat and other fats and fiber

For anyone who's looking to make a little pocket money, you can open a ClickBank account for free, just click on the affiliate link near the bottom of my homepage, and add a link to your emails or tweets. Have the person go through your link to the homepage and when they purchase any book, you'll be paid. Ka-Ching! You won't get rich, but if you want to help people, refer them to the website and get paid something. Who knows what could happen if/when alkalinity goes mainstream!

So with regard to protein powders, word to the wise, don't assume they are harmless or chemically free. You really have no way of knowing for sure.

To obtain the final numbers for our Flaxseed Shake we simply add each line together from each of our four food items.

E=127+150+160+90=527 calories

F=81+70+0+0=151 calories   29.4%

total Fat=83+72+0+0=155 calories   30.2%

SF=10+45+0+0=55 cal

Omega-3 = 39 cal

Omega-6 = 13 cal

Omega-9 = 19 cal

TF=0+0+0+0=0

Chol=0+30+0+0=30mg

Na=0+105+780+21=906mg

K=196+NA+NA+1286=1482mg

CHO=23+48+32+94=197 cal   38.3%

f=55+0+0+0=55 cal

s=0+48+32+94=174cal=33.9%

Prot=18+32+112+0=162 cal   31.5%

T=124+152+144+94=514 cal

LOTS of numbers! I know. Two years from now you will have a

complete handle on this. But for right now it scares you. At the beginning you just buy the food items, make the recipe, and divide it up (aliquot it). The numbers are already crunched. From here on, it's just repetition. You will see the same breakdown, just different numbers for different foods. It's ok ☺ .

Chapter Endnote
At the bottom of page 26 my pitcher's contents is 2192g, however, if you add the grams of each item, 907g for 2lbs cottage cheese x2 =1814g, plus 360g molasses = 2174g. This is 18g more, 2192-2174g=18g, because each container of cottage cheese is really 916g, they give you a few extra grams.

Also note that, 1lb=454g and 2lbs=907g, not 908g. This is because 1lb is really 453.6g, which rounds up to 454, but 453.6x2=907g.

You're becoming an expert already!

CHAPTER 6

KEY PROTEIN

Now let's examine some of the numbers for a closer look at the beauty of this shake meal.

Meal? Yes, a meal. On the far right of the previous page are the macronutrient percents, percent macros. What are they?

Fat = 30.2%
Carbs = 38.3%
Protein = 31.5%

38.3 30.2 31.5, or in whole numbers, 38 30 32.

Recall from the NCD book how we calculate it:
fat cals over Total cals = 155/514 x100 = 30.2%
carb cals over Total cals = 197/514 x100 = 38.3%
protein cals over Total cals = 162/514 x100 = 31.5%

Note also, that there are two percent fats. One using "Calories from Fat" on the nutrition facts label, noted as "F", and the other using "Total Fat in grams" from the nutrition facts label. They are about the same, 151 and 155, and when you crunch them you get 29.4% and 30.2%, about the same.

The carb percent of this meal shake is 38.3%. A bit lower than our target of 40% but that's because there's sugar in this meal and it's also a liquid meal. So, for a shake, a liquid meal, you don't want to go over 40% carbs, and better to keep it a bit under.

While we're at the carbs, let's look at the sugar. The NCD recipes aim at keeping the sugar calories to <100, less-than 100.   This would mean that the percent sugar of the meal is <20%. See how I did that? Meals are 500 calories, 100 over 500 = 0.2 x100 = 20%.

This shake is 174 calories of sugar. Many of you are thinking, WOW, that's a lot of sugar. It is but it isn't. Look closer. 174 calories of sugar over 514 total calories x100 = 33.9%. This meal is about $1/3^{rd}$ sugar. Contrast this with a 12oz can of soda or juice that's 150 calories of 100% straight pure sugar, no fat, no fiber, no protein. This is where the learning comes in. The total sugar is important, but the percent sugar of the entire thing you are eating is equally if not more important – "Glycemic Load" page 188.

A 500-calorie meal with 200 calories of carbs, 40% carbs, and 100 calories of sugar, 20%, is just the right formula to keep your brain from falling asleep and your body from becoming lethargic. If those sugar and carb calories aren't there, you are going to be back in the kitchen or at the vending machine 60 minutes after eating.

Sugar Has A Function – Use It But Don't Abuse It™

Now for our liquid shake, this makes a great way to get proteins fats and carbs into your bloodstream after you just used them all up during your high-intensity workout. I drink half the shake immediately, and then take 20 minutes to drink the rest. If I haven't worked out, then I will drink it gradually over 30-45 minutes while doing errands or at my desk. From experience, I can tell you that I have never had a physiological insulin spike from this shake, not even if I drink the entire shake in 10 minutes. The 34%, one-third sugar, means that the other two-thirds is fat, protein, complex carbs, and fiber, all of which slow down the glycemic load of this shake meal.

There are two other shakes that I see people making that the NCD does not recommend.

#1. The high-fruit high-carb soy/almond/rice milk shake.

Well, we already know that soy milk and almond milk and all the other "milks" are not used in the NCD. We use raw milk, or a good-quality paho milk, pasteurized homogenized milk. Soy is high in plant estrogens and almonds are eaten as raw almonds, unrefined and very close to their original form, just missing their shells. And rice milk, well, where's the protein in rice? Unless they artificially fortify rice milk with protein. The NCD avoids artificial ingredients and manufacturing whenever possible.

This fruit and soy/rice/almond milk shake may contain a little plain yogurt, but most of the time not. Thus, making this shake high glycemic. I would estimate 2/3rds sugar or 75-80% sugar. This would cause an insulin spike, depending on the amount (total calories) consumed, and the speed of consumption.

Bottom line – It's not a meal. It's missing the 30% protein.

In fact, sometimes they add peanut butter to this high-carb shake. What does it turn into when you add peanut butter? DESSERT! It becomes a carbfat. This is why if you are following any other NON-Number Crunching Plan, you may be in big trouble.

You've got to crunch the numbers to see what you are really eating.

You think you are eating "Healthy" but you are simply eating dessert.[TM]

35% fat with 55% carbs-sugar and 10% protein is dessert, even if it's organic nut butter and fresh banana and blueberries. Sorry.

#2. The protein-powder shake.

Here, the recipe calls for protein, because the maker of the recipe understands that you need protein to be there or else it's a dessert.

This person is at least a step more informed than the person above.

Unfortunately, protein powders are not the way to go. They are manufactured. And even though Nutrabio.com makes an excellent protein powder (see ABC NCD), it shouldn't be consumed daily as part of a meal. I've heard of bodybuilders who are allergic to protein powders because their bodies are so overloaded with the stuff. This is why it's important to rotate your foods. By building a Recipe Repertoire. You've heard of P90X and Muscle Confusion, well, think of dietary confusion.

Dietary Confusion™ – where you continually change what you eat.

Most bodybuilders eat the same ten foods week-in week-out, brown rice, broccoli, chicken breast, tuna, sweet potatoes, eggs, egg whites, steak, berries, and protein powder. Then come Saturday night they eat pizza and beer. Well, as long as you're happy and it works for you. For the rest of us, we have the Number Crunch Diet™. And we have the NCD Hawaiian Pizza! Check it out on YouTube! Subscribe!

No one has ever figured out a way of getting casein and whey protein from food, until now.

LIQUEFIED NONFAT COTTAGE CHEESE™

78% PROTEIN – You heard it here first.

Nonfat Greek yogurt is 76% protein, which is good, but it has a mild sour taste, whereas nonfat cottage cheese is fairly neutral. I use greek yogurt in the NCD Pumpkin Cheesecake™ with a crushed almonds, walnuts, and dates pie crust. Another reason I don't use greek yogurt is because most brands have "live active cultures" so you have to be careful about how much you eat. One cup every day would likely be too much. Plus it's more expensive.

Anyway, the reason greek yogurt has become so popular is because of it's high-protein, but lucky for you, you've found a better way!

CHAPTER 7

The Numbers!

The NCD Flaxseed Shake™ is simple, four ingredients. But its amazing benefits are…are…well, there's just so many that it takes 46 pages to write! I am proud to say that this is the longest recipe in the history of the world – Because It's The Most Beneficial.

Moving on with our percent macros, we have 30.2% fat, 38.3% carbs, and the last one, 31.5% protein. This is why it's a meal. A Number Crunch Diet meal. Without that 30% protein, you are moving towards dessert. Higher protein and less carbs and more fat, means you are heading towards the low-carb ProFat Atkins diet. And as explained in the *ABC Water and the Number Crunch Diet*, this strategy only works for a while, as one day your carb cravings and urges are going to overtake you and boom!, you begin a backward trek to where you originally started.

I encourage you to purchase a copy of *ABC Water and the Number Crunch Diet* as it will explain in full detail why the low-carb and high-carb diets are not going to get you to where you want to be in the long term. They might, but for many they don't, and then you just feel more hopeless about getting control of your body weight, and the clock ticks on.

Take control of the numbers and you Take control of your weight.

This is key for bodybuilders and athletes who are looking to gain weight and muscle. Your coach will tell you to eat more calories, but be careful, those calories may not turn into muscle, and then you have a heck of a time getting the weight off if you don't understand the numbers.

Fiber. This shake has 55 calories of fiber, fantastic! That's 55/514 x100 = 10.7 or 11% fiber. This shake is more than 10% fiber. In fact, it's almost half the RDV recommended daily value of 30g. Okay, did you calculate it? I gave you two different units of measure in that last sentence, 55 calories and 30 grams. Fiber is a carbohydrate, so the conversion is x4. Going the other way, from calories to grams, it's /4, divide by 4. So, 55/4=13.75g. Half of your RDV of 30g of fiber per day is 15, so this shake has nearly half your recommended daily fiber intake.

All of you that read ABC NCD surely got that. For the rest of you, BUY THE BOOK!! It will help you more than all the other stuff you spend money on.

Sodium. The NCD likes to keep the sodium, Na, to <1g, or <1000mg. Recall that the < sign looks like an L for less-than. Then the other one, > is greater-than. I call these tidbits. I throw them in in hopes that you will learn other things besides diet. The ABC NCD has, in my opinion, many of these tidbit extras thrown in. Bits of wisdom too. Though I'm not claiming to be the real Messiah! Just the Selfcare Messiah, with tried-&-tested Strategies.

So sodium <1000mg, otherwise I find I get thirsty. Which just means you drink a glass of water 30 minutes after the meal if the sodium is 1300mg. If your meal Na is 1700 or 2000mg, expect your baseline blood pressure to go up ten points on the systolic, (top number), by the next morning. Repeated meals of 1500-1700-2000mg will snowball your systolic, until, uh-oh, you have a headache, and surprise, BP 180 over 95. Typically, the NCD recipes do not have this much sodium. When they do, like for example the NCD Beef Dip™, the recipe makes six meals, and you have one per day, and then you don't make that recipe again for six months. Plus, you balance out this high-sodium meal with low-sodium meals, and there are several very low-sodium meal recipes, and many others are <500mg. Cafeteria food and fastfood are loaded with sodium, and not the good kind. So make your own meals and watch your blood pressure go down.

Cottage cheese is a high sodium food, and this is where all the sodium is coming from in this recipe, sadly, sodium phosphate. The Trader Joe's organic cottage cheese has just as much sodium. But, we are under 1000mg, Na=906, and the sodium is not glutamate, MSG, so we're okay.

Potassium (K). This is not normally included in the nutrition facts, so the NCD doesn't usually include it either, however, what's great is that the K in this recipe is high, 1482mg. Why? Because the sugar ingredient is unrefined. Unrefined means that the minerals are still there. So you get to eat them, making them available for your Divine Intelligence to use within your body as it sees fit. The molasses contributes 1286mg of potassium. This is key. Because if you see that the mineral potassium is there and high, then you can assume it's unrefined and that many of the other minerals are there as well.

Refining takes out the minerals. Unrefining leaves them in.™

High potassium on a food label indicates the food is unrefined.™

An editor once corrected my writing, stating that I was using certain words incorrectly. I knew that. Unrefining is not a word. Microsoft underlines it in red, how could I not know? I use these "incorrect" versions of words to get them to stick, to get under your skin, to gnaw at the back of your head, so that the next time you are grocery shopping, you will pick up plain sugar or grade-A maple syrup, and something will spark, Unrefining Unrefining, and you will ask yourself, "Is what I am buying the most unrefined available?"

I just gave away my secret for getting something to stick and become a part of your life. (Hope it will continue to work.)

Aliquoting is also not a word. It's Unique to the Number Crunch Diet. Every company with an original product does this. You create unique words and features that are linked to your product. Bring a birthday cake to your job and six people will have six different serving sizes.   An aliquot is a measured serving, a calculated serving, it's a Number-Crunched Serving.™

Aliquot – a number-crunched serving.™
Aliquoted – divided the whole into number-crunched servings.™

Aliquoting, the new term in dieting.™

So our potassium of 1482 nicely balances out our sodium of 906, and with a high potassium, we can feel comfortable knowing that the other nutrients and minerals are present as well, unrefining.

Cholesterol 30mg, nothing significant. But the NCD doesn't worry about dietary cholesterol.   What!   Why?   Because the liver synthesizes (makes) cholesterol from excess carbohydrates and sugars. Dietary cholesterol in the body accounts for only 40% of your body's total cholesterol. 60%, more than half, of your body's cholesterol is being created by the liver from too much sugar. The NCD says that high cholesterol foods, like eggs, are good for you.

As amino acids are the building blocks of all your proteins and enzymes, cholesterol is the building block for all your steroid hormones. So rather than take steroids, eat eggs.

Saturated Fat. The NCD doesn't worry too much about this. We need it. But not a complete diet of saturated fat. All I am saying is, the media makes saturated fat out to be bad, because the average person is consuming 50% of their fats as saturated fats. But if you follow the NCD Dietary Fats Explained™, your saturated fat intake will be <30%. No need to dwell on saturated fat. This shake has 55 calories of SF. How many grams is that? Fat grams to calories is x9. Going the other way, then divide by 9, so 55/9=6 grams of saturated fat per shake. No cause for alarm. Pork ribs and nonlean beef and dairy have SF, so that's where you need to pay attention.

T Total calories at the bottom is 514, and E calories at the top is 527, so a bit of a discrepancy but a pass as far as matching goes. Note that there is no "T" on a nutrition facts label. We have added it to the bottom and calculated it by adding together our three foods, fat carbs protein. In this recipe it's 155+197+162=514. Always do this calculation to verify that your E calories at the top is correct. And you should do this with individual foods as well. You ABC-NCD readers will recall our dry powdered milk example, E=80 and T=80.

So what else? We covered %fat, %carbs, %protein, sugar, fiber, sodium, potassium, saturated fat, TF trans fat is zero, as always, per NCD rules, cholesterol, and total calories. Oh, Omega-3!

Just kidding. I didn't forget. I throw humor in here-and-there to keep you engaged. And to give your mind a break.

Here's where it gets exciting! And yes, I really do mean Exciting! You'll see why at the end.

Each shake has 39 calories of omega-3, 13 calories of omega-6, that's fine, we need some omega-6 as it is essential, we just don't want it from refined corn, soy, sun, and safflower oils, we want it from foods, corn on the cob, frozen organic corn, sunflower seeds, nuts, etc. We don't need to "seek out" omega-6. See ABC NCD. And lastly, 19 calories of omega-9 per shake, also known as OAP, Olives Avocado Peanuts. Omega-9 is a good fat and is included in the NCD, but it's not a "Seek Out" fat. Our two seek-out fats are, Omega-3 Flax and Cod Liver Oil fish fat.

So, 39 of 3, 13 of 6, and 19 of 9. 39 calories of omega-3 is the highest, by far. There is three times as much omega-3 as omega-6, 13x3=39, and twice as much omega-3 as omega-9, 19x2=38. So, do you see why you should be eating flax seeds? It's THEE source in the diet of all the foods available with the most amount of omega-3. And the NCD Flaxseed Shake Recipe™ is your way of consuming them. Jumper Publications & Media – from Advice to Results.

I make these plugs for my publications because I was up to my ears with advice from books and magazines and on television, with no real answers for exactly how to do that advice. So I came up with my own methods, or protocols. I hope you can appreciate how unique, simple, and loaded with nutrition this recipe is. And 30% protein with no protein powder! People will say, "That's impossible!" "You have to use protein powder to get that amount of protein, or egg whites." Trust me, and everyone else that's tried it, don't eat raw egg whites. Never mind, go ahead and try it!

So our 39 calories of omega-3 makes up 25% of the fat of this shake. The numbers are, 39/155 x100 = 25%, where 155 is the total number of fat calories. The entire shake is 7.6% omega-3 fat, 39/514 x100 = 7.6%. Our 39 calories of omega-3 is 4.3 grams of omega-3, 39/9=4.3g. (Fat grams to calories = x9. Going the other direction, fat calories to grams = /9.)

If you buy omega-3 eggs, chickens that have flaxseed added to the feed, you'll be paying about $3 for a dozen nonorganic eggs. This is double the price of regular eggs, and all they do is add flaxseed to the chicken's diet. These eggs have 225mg of omega-3 per egg. Your shake has the equivalent of 19 of these eggs, 4300/225=19. If you've read ABC NCD, then you know that 4.3g is 4300mg.

Your flaxseed shake is $1/20^{th}$ of a pound of flax seeds. So if you had one shake per day, for three weeks, then skipped a week, by the end of the year you will have consumed TWELVE pounds of flax seeds. That would be equal to 1 Kg of omega-3 fat!!!!!!!!!!

Yes, 1 kilogram or 2.2 lbs, or 1,000,000mg, or 4444 omega-3 eggs.

39 calories omega-3 per shake times 20 shakes per pound times 12 bags (pounds) a year = 39x20x12=9360 calories of omega-3 per year, divided by 9 = 1040 grams per year, divided by 1000 = 1.04 kilograms Kg of omega-3 fat per year. There are 454g in one pound, so 1040g/454g=2.3lbs. That's 2.3 pounds of omega-3 fat per year. Your body will be quite happy with that. No deficiency. No dry skin. No countless other biological problems.

CHAPTER 8

NCD FSR Variations™

Now before I move on to the two variations of this shake, I regret to inform you that Bush Creek Organic Farms, the maker of this beautiful flaxseed, is no longer in business. I think they are selling their flax seeds to Arrowhead Mills. In the ABC Water book we talked about "voting with your dollars". You see, if you don't vote for these good farmers, they will disappear. And then one day, all we have for food are cereals, margarine, soft drinks, and ice cream. I'm serious. You need to seek out good companies and support them. The healthfood store, organic food, raw milk, organic flaxseed, independent researchers! If you don't give them some of your food-budget money, they won't be around in the future.

So I purchased 17 bags of Arrowhead Mills Organic Golden Flax Seeds, 14oz for $2.99. Great price, and the shipping is free if you spend $49, so 17x$2.99=$50.83. Bob's Red Mill sells the same thing in the 16oz size, but they also sell them ground. Don't buy them already ground, because why? The "U" shape of the fatty acids of omega-3 and fish oil DHA and EPA are very unstable. You grind them and eat them immediately. I will store my ground flaxseed 1-2 days in a sealed airtight container in the refrigerator, but not 4-5 days. Fish, eat it the same day you catch it.

The website is www.vitacost.com. I like this company already.

Whichever brand you buy, the amount is still 23g per shake.

NCD Maple Shake™

For the maple shake you are just going to substitute 275g of grade-B maple syrup for the molasses. Grade B is less refined than grade A, or light amber, and it will therefore have more minerals. I purchase mine at Trader Joe's and it's TJs brand, 32 fl oz, 1 quart, 946mL, for $16.99. But the price of maple syrup keeps going up, so what does that tell you? It's a valuable product.

Now, you will notice that the front label doesn't say how many grams. It lists the product by volume, 32floz, 1qt, 946mL milliLiters. So I have figured out the grams for you.

60mL = 78g

Should you ever encounter a product that doesn't list their food by weight, you will have to do some measuring to figure it out. But the NCD recipes have it all done for you.

So my TJs 100% Pure Maple Syrup Grade-B label reads:
1/4cup 60mL
servings per container = 16 (32oz ÷ 2oz ¼cup = 16)
E=200cal
F=0
total Fat=0g   0%
SF=0g
TF=0g
Chol=0mg
Na=5mg
CHO=53g x4 = 212 calories   100%
f=0
s=53g x4 = 212 cals
Prot=0g   0%
T=212

This product is also from Canada. Try to pick places where things are grown in the-middle-of-nowhere, Hawaii, Alaskan Salmon, North Dakota flax seeds. While driving up the I-5 freeway through

Central California, I noticed something I've never seen before. Several of the orchards had plastic tents over the crops. Dust, dirt and pollution falling on the crops is making them sick. Sadly whenever it rains, the first rain is full of dirt, almost like mud. Your car gets covered in dirt. Then the second day of rain it's cleaner, and the third day of rain is clean rain. So, look at the big picture when selecting foods. If air pollution is bad for people, it's bad for plants too. Coastal areas tend to be cleaner, and rural areas.

So our 275g of maple syrup gets added to our Ninja in place of the 360g of Plantation-brand blackstrap molasses. This means our batch of eight shakes will be 85g less (360-275=85). Dividing by eight, 85/8=10.6, so each shake will be about 10-11 grams less in weight when you go to aliquot it. So, for the molasses shakes you poured 274g into each of the eight 32oz glass jars, for the maple shake you'll pour 263g.

If you weighed your Ninja pitcher empty, then you can always weigh the Ninja pitcher with the NFCC-maple-syrup, and subtract the weight of the empty pitcher to get the weight of your shake batch. Then divide by 8 to get the grams per serving that you will pour. I posted on my refrigerator the weight of my empty Ninja pitcher with lid and it's 1137g. So I just weigh the entire pitcher with contents, subtract 1137, divide by 8 (servings), and that's my number, the number of grams I pour into each jar.

Each shake will have 34g of maple syrup.
E=88
Na=2
CHO=93
s=93

The CHO for the molasses is 94. So the maple syrup will result in essentially the exact same macro percents, 38 30 32, rounded off.

There's no point in crunching it all again. Just substitute 275g of maple syrup for the molasses and aliquot it into 8 servings of 263g. Oh, and Party On Down! Because this tastes delicious! No Kale!

The TJs maple syrup comes in plastic, and if you are a NCD reader then you are a professed and committed Plastiphobe. So I transfer my maple syrup to a one-quart one-liter glass amber bottle using a funnel, and then refrigerate it so that it lasts a long time without degrading, and since I use clean sterile technique when transferring it, I am assured of no bacterial or mold growth.

The 275g of maple syrup is equal to about 212mL. The container is 946mL, so 946/212=4.46 or 4.5. You can make 4.5 batches of this shake per 32oz container of maple syrup. I typically have this maple shake about once a month. So by the end of the year I've consumed about 2½ quarts of maple syrup. You will have no cravings for pancakes with syrup if you follow this protocol.

Your body doesn't want the pancakes, as it's just refined flour. What it wants are the minerals in the maple syrup. Unfortunately, if you eat pancakes at a restaurant you get ZERO minerals as maple syrup is way too expensive so they use pancake syrup, which is just HFCS and maple flavoring. Just like the little peel-off packets of strawberry jam is just sugar and red food dye. Read the label the next time, there's no strawberries in the ingredients, but they're allowed to call it strawberry. Go figure.

Word of warning. In the beginning when you drink this maple shake, your body will recognize the nutrition and say "More More Faster Faster". You are likely deficient in tree sap nutrients. Drink it slowly over 30-45 minutes so that you slow down the glycemic load. As time progresses and you've had say 2+ quarts in 12 months, then you won't feel that urge to drink it so fast.

Do you remember the following from page 159 of the ABC NCD?

What if much of the food you eat over and over again, and overeat, what if, your body's searching for something it needs? Well, not "what if", THAT'S EXACTLY WHAT'S HAPPENING.

Your eyes will see with new insight and you'll be a changed person after you read the book. A better person. A more informed person.

NCD Honey Shake™

Like molasses and maple syrup, honey is so good for you. It's a God food. Made by bees, not man. But there are better brands and kinds than others. I buy Trader Joe's Creamed Honey, 1lb, $4.49. It's 100% North American Clover Honey, Product of USA. The reason I buy it though is because it's UNfiltered and UNcooked. That's what is says on the label, "Unfiltered and Uncooked".

It's Raw Honey. And it's Unrefined.

Our nutrients are present and have not been removed or destroyed.

The honey is hard at room temperature. Hard as a rock. Liquid honey has been heated, "cooked". This liquid honey is now liquid for the life of the product. It's permanently changed. Someone I once worked with had never seen rock-hard honey before.

The other honey I sometimes buy is from Smart & Final, and it's Faraon-brand Honey With Comb. It's liquid honey but it has a big stick of the comb in it. The comb is delicious, not sweet, just chewy and fun to eat. I don't eat the comb alone as it's covered in the liquid honey, but I add it to the shake, (Ninja pitcher), and some of the pieces don't blend so there are a few bits of chewy honeycomb pieces in the shake.

The amount is the same for either honey you use. Add 232g of honey to your Ninja pitcher instead of the molasses. The raw hard honey may not blend smoothly, that is, some of the honey may fall to the bottom and not be blended into the shake. I am still trying to figure out how to prevent this from happening. So, what I do is, add the 232g to a glass bowl and microwave it for 30 seconds, then add it to the Ninja pitcher. I don't like doing this as it "cooks" my raw honey, but it's very minimal, and 30 seconds is just enough to soften it to a thick liquid. The honey will also soften to a liquid if you leave it in a warm area, (near a window on a sunny day). But until I get the hard chunks of honey to blend thoroughly, I am using the 30-second microwaving to soften it some. It doesn't get hot, it just softens it to a thick pourable liquid.

My TJs honey reads:
1T 21g
servings ~22 (it's a 454g container, so 454g/21g=21.6 servings)
E=60
F=0
total Fat=0   0%
SF=0
TF=0
Chol=NL (not listed, but cholesterol is only found in animal foods)
Na=0
CHO=17g=68cal   100%
f=0
s=16g=64cal
Prot=0   0%

Again, it's a 100% sugar food, like molasses, like maple syrup.

Each shake will have 29g of honey, 232g/8servings=29g.
E=83
CHO=94
s=88

Our CHO is 94, same as for the molasses. So we are not going to crunch the full recipe. Just substitute 232g of honey for the molasses and your macros are the same, 38 30 32. Then, 360g-232g=128g/8=16g, use 16g less per aliquot, 274-16=258g per pour.

	per shake	per batch	per pour
NCD Molasses Shake™	$2.82	360g	274g
NCD Maple Shake™	$3.00	275g	263g
NCD Honey Shake™	$2.81	232g	258g

If you use regular milk instead of raw, the price drops by 75 cents per serving, so closer to $2 per shake. But you miss out on the raw proteins and better probiotics. You won't find this much nutrition anywhere for $3. And with 4.3 grams of Omega-3 freshly ground!

CHAPTER 9

NCD HAWAIIAN PIZZA™

Woohoo! You're going to love this! Hawaiian Pizza has been around for decades, so there must be something to it. A friend of mind told me his culinary instructor said that when a dish doesn't work out, he adds his secret ingredient. It was sugar. I say, when a dish doesn't work out, add Bacon! I'm not a huge fan of pork, but I am pro-pork if it's good quality. And there is good-quality or better-than-average pork out there.

So this recipe makes 6. You, of course, can double it and make 12. You will need 5 different ingredients and 8 total items. Starting from the bottom up, we have:

1. pita
2. spaghetti sauce
3. pepper jack cheese
4. canadian bacon
5. pineapple

But, you have to buy the right items or it won't taste the same. Recall from the ABC NCD, how someone tried to make this pizza without the recipe and it "wasn't the same" she said.

1. Whole Wheat Pita Bread
Trader Joe's market, TJs brand, 12oz 340g, 6 pitas per bag, $1.69. Ingredients: 100% whole-wheat flour, water, sesame seeds, wheat

gluten, yeast, salt, distilled vinegar. Nothing too weird. It all sounds like food to me. But you are no doubt looking at that wheat gluten.

Gluten Sensitivity. This is a real thing. I've known a couple of people with Celiac Disease, and they would break out in rashes from the allergic inflammatory reaction to the protein gluten found in wheat. Now I am not a doctor, nor do I play one on the internet, but a doctor is not really a health expert. Doctors are disease identifiers and disease treaters. This is what they are trained to do. If a doctor starts using his own protocols for treating people, he can lose his license. And if he cures people using protocols that aren't approved by the medical board, then he's in big trouble. He becomes a threat to the system.

So we need to rethink and redefine in our minds what a doctor is and is not. Your standard everyday doctor is not really knowledgeable about health and doesn't really understand the root root causes of things. He may understand the first root, but there are second and third roots further down that are the real problem.

In looking at the images of inflamed colons and Crohn's Disease colons and Irritable Bowel Disease colons, I can't help but think – Parasites.

I'm going to tell you what I do to maintain my body parasite-free, and if you've read ABC NCD then you know that pet owners are often carrying around the same parasites as their pets. It's just too hard not to. Best advice, no pets.

When I studied parasitology at Cal State L.A. and during my internship at Smithkline Beecham Clinical Lab, intestinal parasites were the most common. The Hook Worm would make your skin crawl. What do you think that worm does with those hooks? It locks on to the wall of your intestine. Then what? It lays eggs in that wall. Gross. But look at those nodules on the colon walls on the internet. Parasites don't kill you, they live with you, they live off you. They cohabitate. They steal your nutrients for themselves, but worse, they go to the bathroom in your colon. Hence, allergic reaction. Any time I see an inflammatory-skin response or eczema, I think toxins, excrement from worms, or mycotoxin release from yeast and fungus, or bacterial toxin release. Something in your body is reacting to something. And it's likely to be coming from inside your colon.

For this reason, I take two measuring teaspoons, 10mL, of Green Black Walnut Hull tincture every-other Sunday. This is my anti-parasite maintenance program. Recall that I take one or two capsules a week of Oil of Oregano as my anti-yeast, anti-fungus, anti-mycoplasma insurance plan – see page 175 ABC NCD for the kind I recommend.

You can purchase the GBWH at www.drclarkstore.com, currently $26.99 for the 4oz bottle. The active ingredient in the green hulls of the black walnut is Juglone, and it has to appear green when you take it. This is the only website on the internet that understands this. If it's not green when you go to take it, it will make you vomit. However, if it's green, then it's fresh and not oxidized and it goes down fine. DrClarkStore.com guarantees that the product will be green when you receive it or they will ship you a new bottle. This tincture is also 57% GBWH, high potency.

This website is based on the book, *The Cure For All Diseases*, by Dr. Hulda Clark, PhD. Her expertise was pollutants and parasites. It was fifteen years ago that she wrote her book. Today, the information that she discovered and wrote about, trace chemical pollutants being found in our body products, in our foods, in vaccines, in everything, all started with this person's research. Her books have been translated into ten different languages, so clearly, there are people all over the world interested in her discoveries and conclusions.

But the other half of her expertise that we don't hear about, is Parasites. The mainstream has picked up on pollutants, but that was only half the picture. What about parasites mainstream? Well, the mainstream avoids anything that is a bit disgusting or dirty.

Apparently, the media viewers are so pure and clean that we can't talk about parasites. That's too gross for them. And certainly not urine pH. Yuck. Give me a break. The average everyday person is far from being a saint and clean as the pure white snow. Maybe back in the 1950s, but not today.

Regardless, parasites, urine pH, this is all biology. And if you pretend you don't use the bathroom to take care of your biology, then you are not telling the truth. Paying some attention to these things and learning about them and understanding them, well, that's when you are likely to become clean and healthy. The first thing I think of when I see someone with dark circle around their eyes, is parasites. They're out there. So, become aware of them. Living in California, most people never remove their shoes when they enter their homes. Whatever was on the bottoms of their shoes is now on their carpet, floors, sofas, pillows, and it just keeps traveling. But worse, are all those guys wearing flip flops. Yes the ladies like it, but the soles of your feet absorb things, and street dust and dirt is everywhere. I've seen people with flip flops walk into a public bathroom, or go through airport security in bare feet.

So, step one is to do the parasite cleanse, DrClarkStore Para-Cleanse 3, $39.77 for one bottle of the GBWH 2oz, 100 caps of cloves, and 100 caps of wormwood, male fern. The kit comes with the instructions. I've done this cleanse, and I may cover this in full detail later, or in a separate publication, as there are some do's and don'ts, and you have to aliquot the bottle of GBWH into vials otherwise it will turn black by the following Sunday. But if you have ANY digestive or gastrointestinal issues, start with this parasite cleanse, because in my opinion, your problem, the root root of your problem, is Parasites.

Good bacteria from raw milk will repopulate your colon and chase out the bad bacteria. So seriously consider raw milk for colon health.

Refined white flour and water are used to make paste in grade-school classes, so it will do the same thing within your colon.

CHAPTER 10

The Macros

Yes, that aspect of selfcare really needs its own section of a book because I just touched the surface of my protocol, and being parasite-free is super important, especially for fat loss. If you are aware of pollutants, toxic chemicals, metals, etc., then you need to take that next step and become aware of parasites, and avoid both.

As far as gluten is concerned, I don't have a problem with it. My colon works good. It does what it's supposed to.

Nutrition Facts
1 pita 60g
6 per container (bag)
E=160cal
F=15cal
tF=2gx9=18cal
SF=0.5gx9=4.5cal
TF=0
Chol=0mg
Na=240mg
CHO=30gx4=120cal
f=5gx4=20cal
s=0g
Prot=7gx4=28cal
T=15+120+28=163
15/163x100=9%

120/163x100=74%
28/163x100=17%
74 9 17

This food product is 74% carbs 9% fat 17% protein. It's higher in protein than you would expect for a bread product, but it's not refined much. You can tell because the fiber is high, 5 grams, 20 calories, 20/163x100=12%. These pitas are 12% fiber. Good. I would call it a true Whole Grain.

NCD Whole Grain Rule, the percent fiber has to be double digit.™

If the percent fiber of the bread product is 10% or greater, it's a whole grain, Unrefined. Less-than 10% fiber and it's more refined.

The label also says, No Preservatives, No Artificial Colors or Flavors. See, companies brag that they don't put these things in their food products. Preservatives, Colors, and Flavors, not good.

Other than the wheat gluten, the rest of the ingredients are all foods, 100% whole wheat, water, sesame seeds, yeast (needed to make bread), salt, distilled vinegar.

If you "crave" white-crust pizza, that's okay, in the beginning you may not be able to get your mind around whole-wheat brown crust. TJs has white enriched-flour pitas, same product, but 1g less in fiber and 2g less in protein. No big deal. Just use the white ones for a while and then switch to whole wheat. But if you read the ingredients you will see that they add B vitamins to it, because they got removed during the processing. When you start to think of it in that way, processed out, then enriched back in, your brain will say, "Never mind all that, just get the whole-wheat ones." Remember which YOU you are shopping for. I buy the white ones occasionally. Or, if I do 12 pizzas, I'll do 6 whole wheat and 6 white. Just make the white ones an occasional treat.

2. Organic Spaghetti Sauce with Mushrooms
Trader Joe's brand, fat free, 25oz 709g glass jar, buy one, $2.29.

Ingredients: organic tomato puree, organic diced tomatoes, organic mushrooms, organic sugar (nice, not GMO), salt, organic garlic powder, organic onion powder, organic minced onion, organic basil, organic parsley, organic oregano, organic black pepper.

Is this a great product or what? And $2.29. You would pay $1-2 more for nonorganic at a regular supermarket. The company lists every single spice they use, no secret "spices" on the label. Only the salt is not organic, but I don't think you can certify a dried-up sea bed as organic, so I'd say this product is 100% organic. Plus no preservatives, and no words I can't pronounce. Excellent.

Find a similar product yourself if you don't have a Trader Joe's. But make sure it's fat free, because we are using cheese for fat.

Nutrition Facts
1/2 cup 113g
servings about 6
E=45
F=0
tF=0
SF=0
TF=0
Chol=0
Na=350mg
CHO=10gx4=40cal
f=2gx4=8cal
s=4gx4=16cal
Prot=1gx4=4cal
T=44cal
91 0 9
91% carbs 0% fat 9% protein. Plus a serving of RED. Excellent.

3. Organic Pepper Jack Cheese
Trader Joe's brand, 8oz 227g, $5.99. I have switched to buying First Street brand at Smart and Final, 5lbs for $13.49 = $1.35 for 8 ounces, 78% less money (but not organic). And you have to vacuum seal the leftover cheese so that it doesn't spoil and get

thrown away. Ingredients (TJs): organic pasteurized milk, cheese cultures, organic red and green jalapeños, sea salt, vegetable enzymes. Standard cheese ingredients, milk, salt, enzymes.

Nutrition Facts
1oz 28g servings 8
E=110cal
F=80cal
tF=8gx9=72cal
SF=5gx9=45cal
TF=0
Chol=25mg
Na=180mg
CHO=0
Prot=8gx4=32cal
T=112cal

The F fat-cal number of 80 seems more accurate than the tF total fat in grams number of 72, so I am using the 80+32=112. One-sixth of 8oz 227g is 1.3oz 38g so we need to multiply our nutrition facts label by 1.35 to reflect our serving amount per pizza.
E=149
F=108
SF=61
Chol=34
Na=243
Prot=43
T=151

4. 3 packs of Healthy Canadian Style Bacon

Trader Joe's market, Celebrity brand, 6oz 170g, $2.49 each, product of Canada. For some reason, Canada makes good pork. Safeway used to sell boneless BBQ pork ribs in the freezer aisle and they had almost no fat, all meat, protein. This is rare for pork ribs. They were from Canada also. The other brands of canadian-style bacon don't work as well. Hence, this is a key ingredient, as is the spaghetti sauce, with all those organic spices.

Ingredients. It doesn't say ingredients on the label, it just says "made from pork sirloin hips with natural juices". And it's cured with water, dextrose (glucose), potassium lactate, salt, potassium chloride, sodium phosphate, sodium diacetate, sodium ascorbate, sodium nitrite. Yes, that's a lot of sodiums. But it says it's "50% less sodium, 350mg instead of 720mg", and it has the American Heart Association emblem. So we have, water, sugar, and some sodium and potassium salts, and a nitrite. If you wanted to, you could wash them in hot water to remove some of the salts, but I'm okay with it. I don't eat ham or bacon very often.

Nutrition Facts
3 slices 51g
servings per container 3
E=60cal
F=10cal
tF=1gx9=9cal
SF=0.5gx9=4.5cal
Chol=30mg
Na=350mg
CHO=1gx4=4cal
f=0
s=0
Prot=10gx4=40cal
T=10+4+40=54cal
7 19 74

7% carbs 19% fat 74% protein. This is a pretty good source of protein for our pizza, 74%. I am going to recrunch the label because we are going to use 5 slices per pizza, or half a pack, 3oz 85g. 85g/51g=1.67 so we are going to multiply our label by 1.667.
E=100
F=17
SF=15
Chol=50
Na=583
CHO=7
Prot=67
T=91

5. Canned Pineapple Chunks, 2 cans

Any market, Dole or Del Monte brand, 20oz 567g, $2.19. Be sure to buy this when it's on sale to save money, and then when you go to make the recipe you only have to shop for four items. The label says, "all natural fruit, no sugar added, rich in vitamin C, diets rich in fruits and vegetables may reduce the risk of some types of cancers and chronic diseases". You do know why that's true, right? Living plants with living colors, and alkalinity. "Let Food Be Thy Medicine and Let Medicine Be Thy Food" – Hippocrates.

Ingredients: pineapple, pineapple juice.   Pick a brand with just these two ingredients, and not one with citric acid, because if it is derived from corn, it may contain free glutamate.   The canned pineapple from Thailand has citric acid, but the canned pineapple from the Philippines does not.   Check the label.   Tip, the Del Monte brand has the pull-top lid, so superfast and easy to open it.

Nutrition Facts

1/2 cup 122g

We are going to use 1/3 of the can per pizza, so, 567g ÷ 3 = 189g.

189g/122g=1.55 so we are going to multiply the label by 1.549.

E=70x1.55=108

F=0 SF=0 TF=0 Chol=0 no fat, no cholesterol

Na=0 no sodium

K=150mgx1.55=232mg of potassium, as we expect in fruit

CHO=16gx4=64calx1.55=99cal

f=1gx4=4calx1.55=6cal

s=15gx4=60calx1.55=93cal

Prot<1g (no protein)

T=99

100 0 0

100% carbs 0% fat 0% protein. Now, this item is going to be separated into two parts. The chunks go on top of the pizzas, and the juice is your dessert. You can have the juice straight, for a delicious, sweet, pineapple taste, or, you can add an equal part of water to it, or, you can pour the 2.3 fluid ounces of pineapple juice (per pizza serving) into your 32oz glass drinking container and top it with 30oz of water and carry that around with you and sip on it.

This juice that you will drain off from the canned pineapple tastes wonderful! It's a great dessert treat! It's not like the pineapple juice you would buy in a 64oz carton. Dessert doesn't always have to be cakes, cookies, and ice cream. Plus, you can have this 2.3 fluid ounces of pineapple juice and not feel guilty because it's good for you. It's real juice from the fruit. And a serving of Yellow.

The numbers for our pizza with the 2.3floz of pineapple juice are:
E=160+45+149+100+108=562
F=15+0+108+17+0=140
SF=5+61+15=81
Chol=34+50=84
Na=240+350+243+583=1416
CHO=120+40+7+99=266 (minus 34 fiber = 232)
f=20+8+6=34
s=16+93=109
Prot=28+4+43+67=142
T=548
T minus the fiber = 548-34 = 514
The macros are 48 26 26. With the fiber subtracted they become 45% carbs 27% fat 28% protein. This is a bit more carbs than you may want to have, but it's very macro balanced overall, 45 27 28. Plus, if you take the "dessert" and add it to the 32oz jar and drink it with 30oz of water over 2 hours, then the pizza alone is 41 29 30. Or, you can have the pizza alone with no juice for dessert, and just save the juice for your FFS or HFFS, or the NCD One Fruit Meal, see page 187 of ABC NCD.

The pizza alone is:
E=524
F=140
CHO=229 (minus the fiber carbs = 195)
f=34
s=74
Prot=142
T=511
T minus fiber = 477
The macros are 44.8 27.4 27.8, or rounded off, 45 27 28. If you

subtract the fiber, the macros become 41 29 30. The two cans of pineapple have about 14floz of juice, equal to 224 carbcals, divided by 6 = 37 calories. So the juice dessert is 37 calories of carbs, 35 calories of sugar. I am okay with that, as the extra carbs just go to fuel my muscles, however, if you are trying to lose fat, then omit the "dessert". Your pizza will be 41 29 30 and ~500 calories.

Chapter Endnote

As we move forward into the recipes, you will see less spelling out of the numbers 1 through 9, I have to break that rule of grammar to streamline the communication. You will also see fewer commas used when referring to a series of numbers, and you already have caught on that I don't usually place a space between the number and the units of measure, i.e., 25oz and 709g. I am assuming that at this point, you are comfortable with the condensed writing style. In fact, to keep spelling it out in long form, six ounces, four grams, would get irritating to many readers who prefer things "short-and-sweet". If you find yourself getting lost in the numbers, just go back a few pages, or take a break, or just read one chapter a day. It gets easier with repetition. Remember, your goal is to learn one recipe a month and to have twelve recipes in your repertoire at the end of one year. So don't try to master the entire book in two weeks. *12 Changes A Year* – building a NCD recipe repertoire

Also, you may be wondering why the units of measure are given in ounces (oz) and grams (g). Most of Europe, Canada, and other countries use the metric system, but the "Big Boss" USA is still using oz, lbs (pounds), and gallons, so I have to include both. Think of it like being bilingual, "bi-units". It's good for you!

i.e. and e.g.

Technically, these are two different "words". The first means, in other words, or "meaning", or, that is to say. The second one means, for example. Rather than use both, I use i.e., and for e.g. I use the actual words "for example". The use of "i.e." is becoming broader, and its Latin meaning is not strictly applied these days.

CHAPTER 11

Pizza Party!

Step 1
Place a colander in a bowl and add the two cans of pineapple, let drip.

Step 2
Shred the 8oz of pepper jack into a bowl, place it aside.

Step 3
Remove all the canadian-bacon slices from their packages, there are 10 slices per pack, so you will have 30 slices, divided by 6 = 5 slices per pizza. Place 6 slices in a stack and cut the stack into quarters, top-to-bottom, left-to-right, (+), TBLR. You will now have 24 quarter pieces, in addition to your 24 round slices. You will use 4 round slices and 4 quarter pieces per pizza.

Step 4
Place the 6 pitas on a rack, the stainless steel racks that hold the pans, like what you would place cookies on after you remove them from the pan, "cookie racks". I use the racks that come with my toaster oven. I place 2 pitas on each rack. My toaster oven is big and it works perfectly for this.

Step 5
Pour the spaghetti sauce on the pitas. Pour it in the middle of the pita and it will spread to the edges. Use a spatula to remove all the

spaghetti sauce from the jar.   Use the spatula to spread the spaghetti sauce to near the edges of the pitas. Add the cheese, sprinkling it around, dividing it up evenly onto each pizza. Next, place 4 round slices of the ham on top of each pizza, top bottom left right. You will have ham missing in the four corners. Take your quarter pieces of ham and place one piece at each corner. When you are done, you will have placed 4 round slices and 4 quarter pieces on each pizza, and your pizzas will be covered with ham. Place about 12 chunks of pineapple on top of each pizza, and then place the racks with pizzas in the oven.

Bake at 350°F for 25 minutes, then turn off the oven and let them cook 5 more minutes off heat to just right. My toaster oven has grooves for four rack positions. I use the bottom three positions, and then at 15 minutes I exchange the top and bottom racks, leaving the middle one where it is. Perfect.

Slide one pizza off the rack onto a 7.5-inch square cutting board with handle and cut it into quarters, (+), TBLR. Then, slide the pizza from the cutting board onto a plate. The 7.5-inch cutting board allows you to easily transfer the pizza to the plate so that it looks picture perfect. And you will feel like a master chef!

Have a serving and enjoy! Mmm.

Here's the best part.   There will be about one-tablespoon of drippings from the spaghetti-sauce liquid, the ham liquid, and pineapple liquid, on your oven tray. Carefully remove the tray with the liquid drippings and pour a circle of the drippings on top of each pizza. Ah, this is so good!

Allow them to cool and then cover each plate with a "shower cap" plastic food cover, the round ones with the elastic edges, that look like shower caps. Refrigerate. If you don't let them cool before putting the shower-cap covers on, then the moisture will trap inside and make your crust soggy, which still tastes good, but if you want to be able to pick the sections up and eat them, then let the pizzas cool completely before putting the covers on.

Lastly, transfer the pineapple juice from the bowl, just remove the colander and pour the juice into a Sobe bottle using a funnel. You'll have about 14floz of pineapple juice, about 224 calories, say 250. Have a bit more than a quarter-of-a-cup of juice with each pizza for dessert, 2.3floz. Or, have the pizzas alone and save the juice for Fat Free Sunday.

Cost per pizza, $1.69 + $2.29 + $5.99 + $2.49x3 + $2.19x2 = $21.82 ÷ 6 = $3.64. If you buy the cheese in bulk, the price drops to $2.86, and if you buy the pineapple on sale two cans for $3, then the price becomes $2.63 per pizza. Plus you get a serving of red and a serving of yellow. I can make all 6 of these pizzas and have all the dishes washed and put away in 35 minutes, divided by 6 = 6 minutes per pizza. This will be the most rewarding 35 minutes of work you do all day – six minutes per pizza, you have time for that. Follow the steps that I gave you as that's the most efficient way.

You can see a photo of the pizza on my website at www.abcwaterandthenumbercrunchdiet.com. Be sure to subscribe to my YouTube Channel for free videos, and private videos for JPM members.

CHAPTER 12

NCD Roasted Peppers Chicken Pasta™

This one is a slight cheat, but it tastes like a fancy-restaurant meal and it takes only 60 minutes to make 10 meals.

You need 6 different items and 13 total items.
1. chicken serenada
2. spaghetti
3. fire-roasted bell peppers
4. olive oil
5. sundried tomatoes
6. zucchini

1. Chicken Serenada. This is a great product, especially for $5.99. It's got two, big, lean, chicken breasts in it, with bell peppers and onions. Trader Joe's market, TJs brand, 17oz 482g, freezer aisle.

Ingredients: grilled chicken breast (chicken breast with rib meat, water, canola oil, potato starch, sugar, granulated garlic, black pepper, lemon juice concentrate, salt), chino latino sauce [tomatoes, olive oil, water, brown sugar, garlic, soy sauce (water, wheat, soybeans, salt), pineapple juice, scallions, ginger, cilantro, sesame seeds, salt, jalapeño peppers, rice starch], coco caribe sauce (coconut milk, water, cilantro, brown sugar, olive oil, lime juice, parsley, salt, lemon juice, scallions, garlic, red chili pepper, black pepper, rice starch), red bell peppers, yellow bell peppers, onions, poblano peppers.

That was a long list, but did you see anything bad? I didn't. No scary chemical names and most importantly, no Natural Flavors! You would be hard-pressed to find this at a regular supermarket. And it sounds delicious. But why spend half a day making it from scratch when you can buy this and make ten meals in one hour.

Notice, that the two sauces they used are also made from foods.

This is a good product.

You'll need 5 of them.

Half a box 245g
E=260
F=90
tF=10gx9=90 (matches F exactly)
SF=1gx9=9cal
TF=0 (it's a packaged food so be sure to look at the trans fat)
Chol=65mg
Na=510mg (not that much sodium for a frozen-food item)
CHO=14gx4=56cal
f<1g (zero)
s=9gx4=36cal
Prot=28gx4=112cal
T=90+56+112=258cal

90/258x100=35% fat
56/258x100=22% carbs
112/258x100=43% protein

2. Whole Wheat Organic Spaghetti
TJs brand 16oz 454g $1.39, one package. Ingredient: organic durum whole wheat. Terrific. One ingredient. The fiber content is 9.4% but I'm calling it a whole grain. Once it's cooked it's kind of a pale brown color, so if you are not used to eating WW pasta, you won't be able to notice the difference. Ten years ago the WW pasta was very unrefined and raw, but now it's practically the same as white pasta, just cook it thoroughly and it becomes soft and pale

like enriched white-flour pasta.

2oz 56g 1/8th package
E=210
F=15
CHO=41g
fiber=5g
sugar=2g
protein=8g
We are going to use $1/10^{th}$ of the package 45.4g per serving.
E=170
F=12cal
CHO=133cal
f=16cal
s=6cal
Prot=26cal
T=171
78% carbs 7% fat 15% protein, and 16/171x100=9.4% fiber.

3. Fire Roasted Red & Yellow Peppers
TJs brand, 12oz 340g, glass jar, $1.99 each, buy two. Ingredients:
yellow & red bell peppers, water, olive oil, garlic, salt, citric acid.
Looks good to me. It also says on the label, "no artificial colors or
flavors".   Good companies like to brag that they don't put
chemicals in their products.   Because an overabundance of
chemicals in your diet is going to show up somewhere in your
body, sooner or later.

1oz 28g drained, servings about 8, E=15, F=10, CHO=2g, Prot=0.
We are going to use the entire jar, peppers and liquid, so, $1/10^{th}$ of
two jars is E=24 F=16 Na=176 CHO=13 f=6 s=6 T=29.

4. Organic Extra Virgin Cold Pressed Olive Oil
TJs brand, 16.9floz 500mL, dark glass bottle, $5.99. We will use
28g 2T ÷ 10, so, E=24 F=24 SF=4 T=24, everything else is zero.

5. Sun Dried Tomatoes – Julienne Cut
Trader Joe's used to sell these without sulfur dioxide, and organic,

but now theirs is the same as all the other brands. Buy two bags 3oz 85g $1.99 each. Ingredients, sundried tomatoes, sulfur dioxide (for color retention). 85gx2÷10=17g per serving, E=42 Na=24 CHO=34 f=5 s=19 Prot=5 T=39. The label says that it takes 4 pounds of fresh tomatoes to make 3 ounces of dried tomatoes. So, 4lbs x 16oz = 64oz, 64oz ÷ 3oz = 21.3, or 21 to 1. The Mariani brand says it takes 20 lbs of fresh tomatoes to make 1 lb of dried tomatoes, so 20 to 1. That would mean each 17g serving in our meal comes from ~12oz of fresh tomatoes, 17g x 20 = 340g ÷ 454g = 0.75 lb = 12oz. That would mean we are getting about a 12oz pack of tomatoes with each meal. That's a lot, but the ratio is 20:1.

6. Green Organic Zucchini Squash
TJs brand, 1.5lbs, 2 packs, $2.99 per pack. I found it interesting that the organic zucchini was "grown in Mexico" and the nonorganic zucchini was "grown in the USA". Hm. You will need 3 lbs total. No calorie info as it's free, so few calories that it's not worth counting.

Chapter Endnote
In keeping with the brevity style of writing, you will see a few new words, carbfat, profat, netcarbcals, et cetera. Because the Number Crunch Diet looks at foods and meals in a unique and deeper way than is currently being done, this unique and deeper look requires some new words. The word "carbfat" really needs to become mainstream, in my opinion. Most of them you should be able to decipher, netcarbcals = net carbohydrate calories, the carb number with the fiber subtracted.

Here's my challenge to you. The next time you see cake, or any dessert, instead of calling it "cake" call it a "carbfat". Just do it silently in your mind. When you see cake, say, "It's a carbfat." Once you start doing that, you won't want it. Cake is fun. But a carbfat goes straight to your waistline. Just see it for what it really is, and what it really does, and your attitude towards it will change. The appeal will break. You won't want it. The NCD 6th Method for Food Addiction – rename it, call it what it is.™

CHAPTER 13

Prep & Tips

Pre-prep. Thaw the chicken serenade two hours on the counter. Add 2000g, 2L, about 2 qts, half a gallon, of water to a pot. I recently switched to the "ceramic" lined pots and skillet. The box says it's free of PTFE and PFOA, polytetrafluoroethylene and perfluorooctanoic acid, aka, C8. C4 is explosives. Is C8 a close relative? These two chemicals are used to make Teflon. Dr. Clark was big on not using teflon nonstick cookware and recommended using ceramic. I feel it's important to remember people who made highly-significant discoveries, that a decade later is now all-the-rage, yet few people know how it all came about.

I made the switch because nearly all the teflon at the bottom of my pot was gone. Did I eat it? I hope it just got scrubbed off and went down the drain. Word of caution. The minute you notice the teflon coming off, toss it in the trash! Don't wait another 12-18 months, as the teflon is just going to continue to come off. And who knows where it will end up.

These new ceramic pots are great. It's thick, durable, nonstick, and scratch resistant. Thank you Oster!

So, get your water boiling and then we'll start.

Step 1
Break the spaghetti in thirds and add it to the boiling water. Cover

with the lid so that it comes to a boil again, but keep a close eye on it so that it doesn't boil over.

Step 2
Remove the peppers from the jars and chop them on a cutting board into small pieces. Add 14g of olive oil to each jar, replace the caps, shake, and pour it into a large deep bowl. Add the peppers to the bowl. One tablespoon of olive oil is 14g, so no measuring spoons needed. Just place the jar with the peppers liquid on the scale, press on, pour in 14 grams of olive oil. Repeat with the other jar. Cap, shake, and pour them into the big bowl.

Step 3
Remove the lid from the pot and stir your spaghetti. Wash your cutting board and put it away. Remove the boxes and plastic covers from the 5 chicken serenada, getting them ready for the end.

Step 4
Wash your zucchini in hot water and let them drip dry in a colander. If you bought nonorganic zucchini, wash towel dry, wash towel dry, wash towel dry, 3x.

Step 5
Stir your spaghetti again. Get ten of your medium pyrex bowls, place them on the counter and remove all the lids.

The glass Pyrex bowls with the red lids at Walmart come in 4 sizes.
1. extra small = 1cup 236mL
2. small = 2cups 470mL
3. medium – 1qt 4cups 950mL
4. large = 1.75qts 7cups 1.65L 1650mL

Step 6
When your spaghetti is done, pour it into a colander in the sink, keeping it raised, like on a dish rack, or if you can, hold the colander in one hand and carefully pour it. But it's very hot. Just don't rest the bottom of the colander on the bottom of the sink. I put a dish rack in the sink, the colander fits just right, and the

noodles stay protected from sink germs.

Let it drip, and then add the noodles to the bowl with the peppers-liquid-olive oil. Mix. Add the 2 packs of sundried tomatoes. Mix.

Al dente. This is supposed to be the way you cook your noodles, soft on the outside but a little firm on the inside. Forget that French stuff. The reason for al dente is to slow down the digestion of the starch. But you are going to be eating again in four hours so you want your starch now. Plus the chicken, fiber, and oil is going to slow down the starch digestion, so you don't want to slow it down more by cooking your noodles al dente.

I cook my noodles until they are soft and squishy. The package says 10-11 minutes for al dente, I boiled mine 30 minutes. My digestive system is going to have plenty of work to do, it doesn't need to work overtime digesting partially-uncooked pasta.

For the more down-to-earth chefs, someone I was cooking with once, said that the spaghetti is done if you take a noodle, throw it at the wall, and it sticks. If it falls off, it's not done yet. So for funzies we did it. She was serious, and as it turns out, it's a reliable way to test for doneness. Or, you can put a noodle in your mouth, let it cool off a bit first, and test it that way. But record the time, so that the next time you make this recipe, you just set a timer and cook it X number of minutes and you're done.

Aliquot the spaghetti-peppers-tomato mixture into the ten bowls, evenly. Just eyeball it.

Step 7
Using a V-Slicer, the thick-slice side, slice off the end of the zucchini into the trash, and then slice zucchini directly into your ten bowls. Keep doing this until you have sliced up all the zucchini into your bowls.

Step 8 – last step
Take one tray of the chicken and cut the double breast in half in the

tray, then place one breast in one bowl and the other breast in the other bowl. Divide up the peppers and sauce evenly between the two bowls. Repeat four more times. You will now have ten bowls of spaghetti-peppers-sundried-tomatoes, zucchini, serenade chicken breast. Place the lids on the bowls. Holding each bowl firmly, invert 3x to mix the liquid around a bit. Refrigerate.

Time to Eat!
Remove the lid, place the bowl in the microwave, press 2 minutes, then 1 minute, then 30 seconds. Or you can cover it with a paper towel and press 3:30.

This tastes fantastic. But let's look at our numbers!

E=260+170+24+24+42=520cal
F=90+12+16+24=142cal
SF=9+4=13cal=1.4g we don't need to worry about Sat Fat
TF=0 always zero, so you are not going to see this anymore
Chol=65mg again, cholesterol is not a concern on the NCD
Na=510+176+24=710mg 7/10ths of a gram of sodium, fine
CHO=56+133+13+34=236cal -27 fibercals = 209 netcarbcals
f=16+6+5=27cal
s=36+6+6+19=67cal
Prot=112+26+5=143cal
T=142+236+143=521cal
T-f=521-27=494cal

The macros are 45.3   27.3   27.4. The macros with the fiber subtracted are 42.3 28.7 28.9 or 42 29 29. I'm good with this.

The price is a bit higher, $5.99x5 + $1.39 + $1.99x2 + $5.99x0.06 + $1.99x2 + $2.99x2 = $45.64 ÷ 10 = $4.56 per meal. The 2T of olive oil is 0.06 of the bottle. You would likely pay $15 or more with tax and tip at a restaurant. Plus this is way better for you. Each serving has almost 5oz of zucchini, white and green, plus the red and yellow peppers, and 17g of dried tomatoes, from 12oz of fresh tomatoes. And no chemicals or Natural Flavoring. There's a picture of it on the website so go there and check it out!

CHAPTER 14

NCD My Favorite Breakfast™

This breakfast should become your "go-to" breakfast. You could have it every day, or at a minimum, make this once a month. The recipe makes 12. There are three small variations to it so you can mix it up . You will need 8 different items and 9 total items.

1. jumbo eggs
2. egg whites
3. ground beef
4. ketchup
5. bread
6. peanut butter
7. jam
8. oranges

Variation 1 – omit the jam and orange and have a banana
Variation 2 – omit the orange and have pomegranate juice
Variation 3 – omit the jam and orange and have pomegranate juice

But, of course, you have to know how much of everything so that it comes out 40 30 30 and 500 calories.

1. Jumbo Eggs, one dozen
You can buy organic or regular. I buy the regular ones at TJs for $1.99. E=90 F=50 tF=5gx9=45 SF=2gx9=18 Chol=270 Na=80 CHO=1gx4=4 Prot=8gx4=32 T=86, 5 58 37.

Originally, I calculated T, the total calories, using F, the calories from fat number. But, since F is being removed from the new Nutrition Facts label, I decided to switch over to using tF, total fat in grams times nine. However, this tF number is not very accurate and it's making my T at the bottom not match up with my E at the top. So, from here on, I am dropping the tF number and just using F. You are now familiar with tF, total fat in grams, and how to crunch it into calories, x9, so you're good with that.

Also, the NCD recipes have zero trans fat, so I am dropping that number, TF, from here on. You understand trans fat by now, I am sure. Word of warning. Baja Fresh Express Mexican fastfood restaurant has nice looking, healthy looking meals. But, if you read their Nutrition Facts you will see that several of their menu items have 1-4 grams of trans fat. I was surprised at this because the food looks good, but looks can deceive you.

You've got to crunch the numbers to see what you are really eating.

They also use soybean oil in their fryers. In-and-Out Burger fastfood outlet uses cottonseed oil to deep fry their french fries, and the fry guy tosses the cooked fries in the oil again to reheat them. Just make your own meals yourself and stop consuming things that are making you age and stealing your health, drip by drip.

2. Egg Whites – 32oz 1quart or 16oz x2
Walmart is the least expensive place to buy egg whites, 32oz for $3.88. I get mine at TJs, Papetti Foods brand, 16oz $2.19 x2. Ingredients: 100% liquid egg whites, no added ingredients. It says to use within 7 days after opening, so if you buy the 32oz, you will want to use it up before day 7. This is the nice thing about the 16oz size, the second one may not get opened until next week, so I'm good. 3T 46g E=25 Prot=5g. We are going to use 1/12th of 32oz or 76g 2.7oz per serving, E=41 Na=123 Prot=33 T=33.

3. Extra Lean Ground Beef, 96% lean 4% fat – 2 lbs, 2x1lb
TJs brand, 16oz 454g $4.99 x2. The Nutrition Facts for 4oz 113g is E=130 F=40 Prot=21g. Try to find one that matches this. Most

of the 96% lean 4% fat extra-lean ground beef have the same nutrition facts. We will be using 1/6th of 1lb, 2.7oz 76g E=87 F=27 SF=12 Chol=40 Na=44 Prot=56 T=83, 0 33 67. This beef is 33% fat and 67% protein. So even though it says "4% fat" "96% lean" we can crunch the numbers and see that this is deceptive labeling. But the government regulating agency allows this. This ground beef is really 33% fat, by energy, calories. The NCD never uses ground beef with 7% fat or 15% fat, 93/7 and 85/15. These are too high in beef fat. It has to say EXTRA lean 4% fat 96/4.

4. Organic Ketchup – 24oz 680g
TJs brand, organic tomato puree, organic sugar, organic white vinegar, salt, organic onion powder, organic spices, $1.99. Spices spices, red flag. But it's from a company that I trust and the product is organic, so I will assume no addictive chemicals.

Fruits and vegetables that don't have a peel, like tomatoes, strawberries, lettuce, etc., really need to be organic, as the pesticides get soaked into the surface. You can wash them off with the NCD Nonorganic Washing™ procedure, hot water wash, towel dry, 3x, but if you can buy organic, then do so. This bottle of organic ketchup costs less-than the nonorganic brands.

1T 17g E=15, we are going to use 30g, a bit less-than 2T. But again, no measuring spoons. Just place it on the scale, squirt 30 grams, and that's it. It's so easy once you get into the habit of it. E=26 Na=265 CHO=21 s=14 T=21, 100% carbs, (and sodium).

5. Sprouted Rye Bread – one loaf 24oz 681g
TJs brand, sprouted organic ww berries, filtered water, unsulphured molasses, wheat gluten, sprouted organic rye seeds, organic sunflower seeds, fresh yeast, sea salt, organic sesame seeds, poppy seeds, soy based lecithin, whole caraway seeds, whole dill weed, whole celery seeds, cultured wheat, $3.29. Great ingredients. Lots of seeds. Yes gluten, and yes soy lecithin, but lecithin is actually good for your brain and nerves, but better to get it from egg yolks. Regardless, for $3.29 this is a great loaf of bread. The actual weight of the bread is 704g, so divided by 20 slices makes each

slice 35g.   Our nutrition facts label says each slice is 34g, 681g÷20=34g. We are not going to worry about one extra gram of bread per serving. Just remember that some breads may say "one roll 71g" but the rolls are really 90 grams!

We will be using one slice per meal, 34g, E=90 F=10 Na=140 CHO=60 f=8 s=8 Prot=20 T=90, 67 11 22. This bread is 22% protein. Nice. 8/90x100=9% fiber. But clearly it's unrefined and a true whole grain, or better yet, a sprouted grain.

6. Organic Peanut Butter – 16oz 454g $4.99

TJs brand, I buy the creamy unsalted one, ingredients, organic peanuts. Two words, organic and peanuts. Do you see how the NCD has you choosing foods that are close to their base form? They took peanuts and ground them, just like you would do at home. You don't need all that other "stuff". Store it in the refrigerator and use it within 30 days and you're fine. It also says Product of Canada, hm, that's weird. I thought all the peanuts came from here in my area. So my organic zucchini came from Mexico and my organic peanut butter came from Canada. AMERICA! Wake up. If we are not on our guard, the next generations will be eating 50% of their diet from MONSANTO!

VOTE WITH YOUR DOLLARS

Vote out the bad and vote in the good. Think about every dollar you spend and who it's going to.

Why can't everything be organic?
Why do we need nonorganic food anyway?
Just stop buying it.

Make food choices based on your Internal, instead of your External, and your food choices will change. Divine Intelligence

We will be using 1T 16g of peanut butter per meal, E=95 F=70 SF=9 Na=3 CHO=14 f=6 s=2 Prot=16, 14 70 16. Peanut butter in NOT a protein food, like you hear people say. It's 70% fat. You have to crunch the numbers to see it. Plus 14% carbs and 16% protein. Our sprouted bread is higher in protein, 22%. All nuts, seeds, AND peanuts are fat foods, 70-90% fat calories.

7. Organic Reduced Sugar Strawberry Jam
TJs brand, 15.2oz 431g, $3.49. You will use the entire jar for your 12 meals, 2T per meal x12 = 24T. If you want to use sweeter jam, the regular ones, then use 1T, or half. Ingredients: organic strawberries, organic sugar, water, fruit pectin, calcium chloride and citric acid. The blueberry jam says organic blueberries. Using organic strawberries and organic blueberries costs money. This company is trying to give you a good-quality product for your money. Support Them.

The nutrition facts say, 1T 18g E=30. Regular jams will say 1T E=50. Our 2T 36g serving will be E=60 CHO=56 s=48 T=56, 100 0 0, 100% carbs. But it's going to make our meal FUN!

8. Oranges – 4lb bag of small oranges
TJs market, 10 oranges, $2.99. 4lbs is 1.82Kg = 1820g÷10=182g per orange. The label says one orange 154g, 11 oranges per bag. If you can find a 4lb bag with 12 oranges, that would be ideal, as you can have one orange with each meal. If you have 10 oranges in a bag, then you will have 5 oranges with 6 meals, so you'll slice the orange and put one wedge in a container in the refrigerator for tomorrow's meal. Or, you can eat the entire 182g orange with the meal and cut back your ketchup by half, from 30g to 15g. Or, you can just eat the entire 182g orange, but just realize that you're getting 15 extra carb calories. For me, it's not a big deal, but if you are trying to lose fat, then you don't want to be taking in too many extra carbs than you should. You can also save the extra wedge of orange in the refrigerator and have it as a 15-calorie sugar boost between meals. It's not a big big deal.

If you do have one orange with each meal and your bag has 10 oranges, then you will need a carb for your 11th and 12th meals. This is where Sunview black raisins come in handy. Substitute 18g of raisins for the serving of orange. You can also have the 182g orange with meals 1-5 and 7-11, and then no orange with meals 6 and 12. Again, if you are trying to lose fat, these are your options. If you're active 16 hours a day, or you do cardio and lift weights, then don't worry about it, you're burning calories.

The numbers for this recipe simply work best if your orange is 154g, 12 oranges in a 4lb bag. E=70 CHO=84 f=28 s=56 Prot=4.

Variations

You can omit the jam and orange and have one extra-small banana, 4oz of flesh, about the length of banana flesh that would fit between your thumb and index finger. This is a great way to get that peanut-butter and banana flavor that most of us enjoy. Or, you can have half the banana (2oz) on your bread/toast with peanut butter, and have the 154g orange as well. In other words, you can substitute the 2oz of banana for the 2T of reduced-sugar jam.

2T reduced-sugar jam = 56 carbs
1T regular jam = 52 carbs
2oz of banana = 53 carbs, 46 net carbs with the fiber subtracted
small 154g with peel orange = 84 carbs, 56 net carbs
77g 2.7oz of pomegranate juice = 51 carbs

So, our breakfast has about a 50carbcal serving of jam and about a 50carbcal serving of orange. You can mix them up to keep it interesting. You've heard of "Super Foods", well, pomegranate juice is a superfood, rich in color. Buy the Bolthouse Farms brand, 100% pomegranate juice with nothing else added. The POM brand blueberry pomegranate juice has natural flavor. Bolthouse Farms also has a great carrot juice, and other juices. GO Bakersfield! Bolthouse and Sunview are my local growers and they are great companies. Plus, Bolthouse puts additional information on their labels. Whenever you see a company putting additional information on their label, they are telling you, "We are informed, and we want you to be informed too." Show your support for these caring companies.

CHAPTER 15

Sat Fat & Cholesterol

Think of this breakfast in four parts. The egg and egg white with a sprinkle of curry, turmeric, or cloves. The beef patty with ketchup. The slice of toast with peanut butter and jam. And the orange for dessert. This will satisfy your craving for eggs, and also for a fastfood burger. If you have this mini burger at breakfast, you won't want a burger for lunch. If you have this breakfast every day, then after four weeks you will have eaten the entire 454g 1lb container of peanut butter. Your cravings for peanut butter will be gone. You will also have had 28 slices of bread, so you can look at bread and say, "No, I'm fine." If you had the 4oz banana, that would be 28 extra-small bananas, or if you had the jam and orange, you will have had more than two-dozen oranges.

Do you see how nutrition is going to fill you up and satisfy you?

I hope you can also see how different this is from what the majority of the people are doing. You don't need to reinvent the wheel. The system is already invented for you. Just jump in and begin!

Step 1
Spray a large oval skillet with nonstick organic canola or coconut oil, turn it on to 300°F and add 3 jumbo eggs and 8oz 227g of the egg whites and cover with the lid. Trick. My 16oz egg-white carton weighs 35g, plus the 454g of egg whites = 489g total. If I want to add 227g to the skillet, I can't put the skillet on the scale

and pour 227g. So here's what you can do. The total weight of the carton and egg whites is 489g, minus 227g = 262g. So, pour the egg white into the skillet, then place the container on the scale, if it says 300g, then you know you need to pour a little more into the skillet, then weigh it again, and if it's close to 262g, then you have removed 227g from the carton. Once you've done this a few times it will become instinctive. You'll get a feel for half the container, and then you'll put the carton on the scale and it will read 260 or 265, boom!, you got it on the first try.

I have a bowl that sits on top of one of my scales and I can actually place the skillet on top of the bowl, turn on the scale, it reads zero, and I pour 227g of egg whites into the skillet. Be creative!

When you place the lid on the skillet, set a timer. As a clinical laboratory scientist, we are always setting timers. I've tried dozens of them. I have the Acurite big-digit big-button timer with two heavy-duty magnets on the back. I have two of them side-by-side on my refrigerator. They never move, thanks to the dual magnets. Also, check the beep tone. If it's too loud and piercing, you won't like it. My acurite has a nice normal beep-beep that says calmly "time's up", not "TIME'S UP!!!". Walmart used to sell them but they have different models now. Try amazon.com, or it may be discontinued. Set your timer for 3 minutes.

Step 2
Remove the ground beef from one of the packages and pull it in half, into 8oz and 8oz. Place one of them in a flip-top sandwich bag, then place the sandwich bag with your 8oz beef in a vacuum-seal bag and vacuum seal it. Pull the remaining 8oz of ground beef into three equally-sized mini patties. Place them into your double-sided grill, (the small Sunbeam), and cook your patties on medium. Place one slice of the rye bread in your toaster and start it.

Step 3
Your egg timer is beeping, unplug the skillet and check your eggs for doneness. If they are a bit runny still, then replace the cover and allow them to finish cooking to just right off heat. Your patties

are 3/4ths done, unplug the sunbeam grill and allow them to finish cooking off heat to just right. For me, I unplug it when they are rare, and they continue to cook to med-rare, perfect for my tastes.

Step 4
Grab two small glass pyrex rectangles with the red lids, Walmart, and use a spatula to transfer one egg-with-egg-white serving to each rectangle. Cover and refrigerate. Place the remaining egg-egg-white serving onto your plate. Place one of the patties next to it. Place the plate on the scale, press tare to zero it, and then squirt 30 grams of ketchup on top of the patty. Place the remaining two patties into two extra-small pyrex bowls, place one on the scale, squeeze 30g of ketchup, repeat with the other, cover & refrigerate.

Step 5
Your toast has popped up. Place it on your plate, place the plate on your scale, zero it, add 16 grams of peanut butter, spread it around, then add 36 grams of your reduced-sugar jam. Put the jam and peanut butter away, and quickly wash and dry your double-sided grill and your skillet and put them away as well.

Step 6
Take one orange, slice it onto your plate, sit down, and Enjoy!

This breakfast is so satisfying that you really won't mind the extra work. You'll become more efficient at it the more you make it.

I have this breakfast MTW of each week. So tomorrow and Wednesday, I just make the toast, heat the patty in the microwave, or eat it cold, and the same for the egg. No grill or skillet to wash.

Leftovers.

When you are finished your 12 breakfasts, you will have 8 slices of bread left over. Place them in a stack on the counter. Using your bread knife, saw through the stack about 1¼ inches from the edge, and repeat, sawing through the stack about 1¼ inches from the edge. You will now have 24 "breadsticks", strips of bread, 8 slices of bread cut in thirds. Place them in a container in the refrigerator, allowing them to go stale, hard. I use a white plastic ice-cube container. Try to stagger them and keep some space between them. You will use these breadsticks for the NCD Sausage Pizza™.

Tip. When eating the egg-egg-white portion of your breakfast, slice up the yolk and egg white and mix them together. Soft warm liquid egg yolk is what tastes so good, so coat the egg white with the warm liquid yolk by cutting it up and mixing them together. This can only happen if you cook the yolk to JUST RIGHT, and the 3/4ths doneness off-heat cooking technique should allow you to get it right.

Tip. Find the setting on your toaster so that your toast pops up at just the right doneness. My toaster setting is with the line on the moveable bar at exactly under the "2". Do this and you won't have to keep checking it. And you won't over-toast it either. That black part on the burnt toast is CARCINOGENIC, as are the black grill marks on a hamburger patty. Use medium heat to avoid burning.

The final numbers, using the 154g 5.4oz orange and 2T jam, are:
E=90+41+87+26+90+95+60+70=559
F=50+27+10+70=157
SF=18+12+9=39
Chol=270+40=310
Na=80+123+44+265+140+3=655mg
CHO=4+21+60+14+56+84=239 minus 42 fiber = 197
f=8+6+28=42
s=14+8+2+48+56=128
Prot=32+33+56+20+16+4=161
T=557
T-f=557-42=515
The macros are 43 28 29, using the net carbs they're 38 31 31.

Having had this meal many times, I can say it's just right. No lethargy from too little carbs and sugar, and no insulin spike. Don't worry about the 310mg of cholesterol, you need cholesterol. See ABC NCD for more about cholesterol. Sodium, 2/3rds of a gram, not a problem. Sugar, 128 calories, but that's only 25% of the entire meal, 128/515x100, and you are going to need some sugar to get you out the door to work!

Saturated Fat, SF, RDV, recommended daily value, is 30% of your daily fat intake. If you eat 2500 calories a day of 40 30 30, your caloric fat intake is 750, and 30% of 750 is 225. Therefore, your daily limit of saturated fat is 225 calories, or 25g. Our breakfast has 39 calories, so 39/225x100=17%. This meal has only 17% of the RDV of saturated fat, and yet we ate egg yolk, a beef patty, and peanut butter. For this reason, I am dropping the SF number from here on. It's just not an issue on the NCD. High saturated fat is seen in fatty beef and fatty pork, butter, sour cream, cheese, chocolate, and coconut. The NCD uses lean meats, and when we do have pork ribs, our meal is 500 calories with 150 calories of fat. Just suppose that all of those 150 calories of fat was saturated fat, it would still be under our 225 calorie a day limit. I've included SF up until now so that you could see for yourself, and so that you understand saturated fat. The saturated fat warning applies to people who are eating double cheeseburgers at fastfood outlets day after day. But the good news is, this doesn't apply to you!

Cholesterol is being removed from here on as well. Recall that high blood cholesterol is the result of high blood sugar, and not so much from cholesterol-containing foods. Natural forms of dietary cholesterol are good for you, in fact, they are essential if you want to synthesize the steroid hormones that make you look and feel younger. I haven't read the book, *The Cholesterol Myth*, but I don't need too. I've known it's a "myth" before this book was published. If at some point I do decide to read the book, it will only be to find evidence of the relationship between statin drugs, (taken to lower cholesterol), and Viagra and Cialis prescribed to these same men because now they can't make sex hormones because they lack cholesterol. I know a cardiologist that was taking a statin drug and he came up to the lab in a panic because his cholesterol result was 360. The NCD doesn't buy into prescription drugs, and the NCD doesn't buy into everything the medical system says or proclaims. We think for ourselves, and look to our Divine Intelligence.

Lastly is our pomegranate juice, the 52floz 1.54L bottle from Bolthouse Farms. If you had a 2.7floz ~50-calorie serving instead of the orange, you would have enough servings for 20 meals. If you omit the jam and just have the slice of bread with the peanut butter, then you could have a 5.4 floz serving So, for variety, have 10 meals with 5.4floz of pomegranate juice, 10x5.4=54floz, (they give you a bit more than 52floz), and then for meals 11 and 12, have banana. So instead of the oranges and jam, you'll buy the pomegranate juice and 2 extra-small bananas.

We will also be having pomegranate juice with our breakfast nut meals (TCY-3). So stay tuned for that!

Note, nearly every different brand of oranges has different nutritional facts for a 154g 5.4oz orange. Some brands of oranges have more juice and less fiber. I chose the TJs nutrition facts with the higher fiber, f=7g.

Price per serving is $1.99 + $2.19x2 + $4.99x2 + $1.99x0.53 + $3.29x0.6 + $4.99x0.42 + $3.29 + $2.99 = $27.75 ÷ 12 = $2.31 per meal. That is one nutrition-packed meal for $2.31. And I hope you'll make it "Your Favorite Breakfast" too!

CHAPTER 16

NCD BBQ Chx & PB Choc™

Time for some chocolate! Are you ready!

Now, this meals is going to seem a bit of an odd combination, but that's okay, you just eat it as two parts. Basically, you are having the protein/meal part and then having the carbfat/dessert part.

You'll need five different items and five total items.

1. chicken breast
2. BBQ sauce
3. peanut butter
4. dark chocolate
5. dates

I make this recipe when I have leftover chicken. If my chicken recipe requires 3.25 lbs of chicken, I buy the 6 lb value-pack and with the leftover chicken I make this recipe. I figure, if I am going to boil chicken breast, I might as well do the full 6 lb value-pack.

1. Chicken Breast
Most of the supermarkets have the same lean chicken breast. I might buy it at Food Maxx, or at Smart and Final, just keep in mind that some of them are saturated in as much as 15% sodium phosphate solution. Try to get one that says 1% solution. Read the Nutrition Facts. The Sodium per 4oz serving should be 75mg. The

chicken breast in the 15% solution will say 470mg!!!

Foster Farms is a good brand so I will use their nutrition facts for my numbers, 4oz 113g E=120 F=10 Na=75 Prot=26gx4=104cal T=114, 0 9 91. This chicken is 91% protein and 9% fat. After we boil it, you will see tiny fat droplets in the water, so in my opinion, boiling it turns it into fat-free chicken.

We will be using 5oz raw 3.8oz cooked.

I have spent some time weighing my raw chicken, boiling it, and then weighing it again to find out the raw-to-cooked ratio. Boiled chicken weighs about 75% of that of what raw chicken weighs. This is not the case for grilled chicken. I will go over that in the NCD Chicken Fajita Pita™ recipe. So, our 5oz raw chicken times 0.75 becomes 3.75oz cooked, or 3.8oz.

Put that to memory.

If you want to convert cooked to raw, then take the cooked weight and divide by 0.75. So, 3.75 ÷ 0.75 = 5oz.

NCD Boiled-Chicken Conversions™
Raw to Cooked = times it by 0.75
Cooked to Raw = divide it by 0.75

Our numbers for 5oz raw are E=150 F=13 Na=94 Prot=130 T=143.

2. BBQ Sauce
TJs brand, All Natural Barbecue Sauce, 18oz 510g, $2.49, tomato puree (water, tomato paste), sugar, distilled vinegar, cornstarch, salt, spice, molasses, natural flavor, caramel color, onion, garlic. If you are freaking out, GOOD! You should be. NATURAL FLAVOR is our code word for chemicals that make me addicted to their product. SPICE! Notice it doesn't says spiceS, plural. It just says spice. One spice. I would bet that this one SPICE is MSG. Terrible. For this reason, I am experimenting with making my own BBQ sauce from scratch. It's super easy. You just have to play

around with the different ingredients until you get it the way you want it. My first batch was a little too Dijon mustardy. So until I get it right, I am using this TJs BBQ sauce. The label says, "smoky sweet with just the right amount of kick". Yeah, that flavor kick is MSG. Two tablespoons 34g = 45 calories, we will use 60g, E=79 Na=371 CHO=78 s=71 T=78.

3. Organic Peanut Butter – same as before
We'll use 22g per meal, 22g/32g=0.69, so we multiply our nutrition facts label by 0.69, E=131 F=96 Na=3 CHO=19 f=8 s=3 Prot=22 T=137.

This organic peanut butter is a "Stock" item, as are the sunview black organic raisins, and the 85% cacao dark chocolate bars. I will start pointing out items that are "stock" so you can also consider stocking them. The organic ketchup is always in stock, one in-use and a new one next to it. This way, when you go to make a recipe, you may only need to stop at one or maybe two supermarkets to get what you need.

4. Organic 85% Cacao Chocolate – 100g 3.5oz bars
Green & Black's brand, available at Walmart, but not all Walmarts. Try another walmart if you don't find it. It's a good price, $2.97, for organic dark chocolate. Ingredients: organic chocolate, organic cocoa butter, organic cocoa, organic raw cane sugar, organic vanilla extract, Kraft Foods, made in Poland, 100% Fairtrade compliant. Interesting. Why Poland? Seems like a long way to travel to end up in California. It also says "suitable for vegetarians". It comes from a plant.

12 pieces 40g 2.5 servings per bar E=250 F=180 Na=10 CHO= 15gx4=60 f=4gx4=16 s=8gx4=32 Prot=4gx4=16 T=256, 24 70 6, 24% carbs 70% fat 6% protein. We will be using 3 squares 10g per serving, E=63 F=45 Na=3 CHO=15 f=4 s=8 Prot=4 T=64.

5. Medjool Dates – 16oz 454g $4.49
TJs brand, 2 dates 40g E=110. We will be using 35g E=96 Na=9 CHO=109 f=11 s=95 T=109, 100 0 0, 100% carbs.

CHAPTER 17

Steady Energy

Step 1
To a 20-quart stockpot add two gallons of water, cover and bring to a boil. Use a scissors to cut any visible fat off the chicken breasts. When the water is boiling, add the chicken.

Step 2
Unwrap your dark chocolate bar and break it in half and continue breaking it until you have 30 single squares. This is enough for ten servings, 3sq x10 = 30 squares. Place them all in a container, I use the 12oz glass SKS jar with screw cap.

Step 3
Check your chicken. Remove one breast and cut into it. If it's medium-well with just a faint line of pink in the middle, remove the pot from the heat and use tongs to place the breasts next to your cutting board, allowing them to finish cooking off heat. Wash and dry your pot and put it away. Sharpen your cutting knife. Hold your sharpener in your left hand, arm straight and pointing 45° down at the floor. Now run your knife across the top of the sharpener, then across the bottom, top bottom top bottom top bottom top bottom. That's ten swipes. Wipe the knife. Do this knife sharpening every time you make chicken as it will make slicing and dicing up those chicken breasts fast, easy, and fun!

Your chicken is done and ready to cut.

Place one breast on your cutting board with the thin end on the right and the thick end on the left and cut it from the thin end to the thick end. Just slice and push down, slice and push down, boom boom boom boom. Now, rotate your arm counterclockwise a bit, elbow up, and slice coming back the other way from the thick end to the thin end, slice push slice push slice push slice push. Place a colander in a bowl and use your tongs to transfer the diced chicken into the colander. Dice your remaining chicken breasts. Nice job. For a rookie.

If you were making the NCD Chicken Bowl™ you would add 60oz of this cooked diced chicken to your big deep bowl of rice and beans. This would leave you with about 12oz of leftover chicken.

Grab three 8oz SKS jars with the screw caps. Place one on the scale, add 3.8oz of cooked chicken, press tare to zero the scale and then add 60g of BBQ sauce. Cap & Shake, refrigerate. Repeat twice more. Your leftover chicken made three servings. If you have more chicken left over, just make more servings.

Step 4 – Time To Eat!
Open the jar of barbecue-sauce-coated chicken breast and eat it cold with a fork. Mmm. Place a small dessert bowl on the scale and add 22 grams of peanut butter. Place 3 squares of your dark chocolate into the peanut butter. This 22g of peanut butter and your 3 squares of dark chocolate are…a Chocolate Bar! Enjoy it! It's awesome. So much better than a store-bought chocolate bar.

Step 5 – Medjool Dates, optional
Now the chocolate has theobromine, a slightly weaker version of caffeine, so you are going to feel pumped and full of energy and in a good mood, so you may not want, or need, the dates. But the recipe is crunched with the dates. If you want to lose fat, skip the dates, as it's ~100 calories of sugar. If you did 30-45 minutes of weights this morning, then go ahead and have the dates, your muscles need them. If you are on maintenance calories and you weren't active today, then have one date not two. The label says 2 dates are 40g but in reality 2 dates are 33-37g, so 35g averaged.

The final number are:
E=150+79+131+63+96=519
F=13+96+45=154
Na=94+371+3+3+9=480
CHO=78+19+15+109=221 minus the fiber carbs = 198
f=8+4+11=23
s=71+3+8+95=177 s=82 with no dates
Prot=130+22+4=156
T=531
T-f=508

Macros, 42 29 29, macros with net carbs, fiber subtracted, 39 30 31. Now again, if your goal is fat loss, then no dates. If your goal is muscle size gain and you worked out, then yes, two date. The person who worked out and is looking to gain size can benefit from the 177 calories of sugar. The fat loss goal person will stick with the no dates and 82 calories of sugar. With the no dates, the CHO becomes 112, and T=422, so the macros are 27 36 37, 27% carbs 36% fat 37% protein. This is tweaked towards the low carb, which is an acceptable strategy on the NCD. Recall page 255, "If you want to lose weight a bit faster because you are really motivated, then just omit some of the carbs from a meal, but do it sporadically so that your body doesn't notice you're cutting extra carbs."

40% carbs is a nice steady energy. Dropping it to 30% or below is fine for one meal a day, two at the most. BUT, making all of your meals 30% or 25% carbs is not going to last and you WILL rebound back (yo-yo) at some point in the future. Coffee and diet coke will allow you to keep going, but at some point it will all come crashing down like a house of cards. The NCD is not a "get-thin-quick" scheme. It's a solid mathematical approach to weight management.

When you control the numbers, you control the desired result.

When you cut your carbs to 30 and 25%, your mind becomes fixated on food because your brain is short on fuel and it keeps saying to you, "When do I get to eat, when do I get to eat?"

With the Number Crunch Diet, food is not on your mind. You are satisfied, active, and productive. Then you stop and eat every two to four hours, 250 or 500 calories, just because you know it's time to eat, not because you're hungry and feeling zapped.

That's the whole point of eating every 2-4 hours, so that you AVOID BECOMING HUNGRY.

If food is on your mind, then you are not doing the NCD correctly. Food should not be on your mind with the NCD. You should feel completely satisfied and fine with 40 30 30 meals. My mind rarely thinks about food or when my next meal will be.

Finally, is the price per meal. If you buy the chicken on sale for $2.49 a pound, it crunches to $1.99 a meal. This is $1 below my target of $3 a meal, so it balances out the higher-priced meals. However, this $3 target is going to have to be raised to $3.50 or $4 a meal, because the fastfood joints recently increased the prices of their combo meals by a dollar something, and gas is about to take a big jump in January, so don't hold me to these prices. They are merely a guide so that you get an idea of how nutritiously you can eat when you buy well-chosen products from a supermarket and prepare it yourself. Your goal should be that 100% of your food-budget money is spent on grocery items. No vending machines, no coffee houses, no cafeterias, no fastfood, and no minimarts.

There is one variation to this meal, and that is, instead of the ~100cal of dates, you can have the ~100cal 5.4oz of pomegranate juice. Or you can have one extra-small banana, or one med-Lg orange, or any of the other 100-calorie servings of fruit, 12oz of watermelon, 5.6oz of grapes. At some point, I need to share with you my fruit-serving information, how many grams to weigh out if you want 100 calories of any particular fruit, or if you want 50 calories or 250 calories. Besides the Vegan and the Vegetarian, there are those people who just eat fruit, Fruitarians. You can get all the carb energy you need from plants. So you will see fruit, legumes, and starch vegetables, as the first choice for carbs on the Number Crunch Diet, not grains.

CHAPTER 18

NCD Orange Chicken™

Let's do another chicken, as there's a couple of interesting things in this recipe that refer to things we've previously discussed.

You will need 4 different items and 7 total items. The recipe makes 16. You'll eat 2 the first day, then 3 3 2 2 2 2 = 16 in 7 days, or sometimes I finish them in 10 days. Just to give you an idea.

1. orange chicken
2. rice
3. chicken breast
4. hempseed

1. Mandarin Orange Chicken
Smart and Final supermarket, First Street brand, 22oz 624g, $4.99, freezer aisle, you'll need 4. The chicken ingredients say, breast meat chicken with rib meat, water, unbleached enriched wheat flour (wheat flour, niacin, reduced iron, thiamine mononitrate, riboflavin, folic acid), soybean oil, cornstarch, contains less than 2% of, modified food starch, salt, isolated soy protein, potassium carbonate, dextrose, eggs, spices, whey solids, carrageenan, tricalcium phosphate, sodium bicarbonate.

So where do we draw the line? Which of these are foods and which are not foods? Interestingly, the ENRICHED flour with the added B vitamins has nitrate. Our thiamine B1 has a nitrate attached to it. So this is a bit like our canadian bacon cured in sodium nitrite. The NCD pays attention to Nitrates and Nitrites, but it's hard to omit them completely, this is why we have the "Occasional" rule. The body is designed to eliminate toxins, and that's the good news. But we live in a toxic world, so we have to pay attention to the toxins in our homes, workplaces, bathrooms, kitchens, garages, and do the best we can to limit them.

Any time you see "less than 2% of" on an ingredients label, chances are there's going to be some questionables. Modified food starch, soy protein isolate, spices, carrageenan, are all questionables. Spices, notice that it's plural. Dextrose is glucose. Calcium with three phosphates, fine. Sodium bicarbonate, baking soda, our hero! The cover of the box says "No Preservatives No MSG Added", so that's comforting.

The sauce says, water, sugar, distilled vinegar, soy sauce (water, soybeans, wheat, salt, sugar), modified cornstarch, spice, ginger, garlic, mandarin orange flavor.

SPICE. Now this one is singular. Recall from the ABC NCD that the SPICE called "Accent" has one ingredient, MSG, monosodium glutamate.

NCD SPICE Rule™
If you see SPICE singular, strongly suspect MSG. Spices, plural, could be just spices, or it could have MSG or some other addictive chemical thrown in.

It's hard to know for sure, as we don't have access to the company's files. And they keep all this very tightly capped. Call a food company sometime and ask some specific questions. You will quickly be rebuffed. What are they hiding?

Recall that most organic-food manufactures go out of their way to tell you everything that they can feasibly get onto a product label.
Organic-Food Manufacturers = Disclose
Processed-Food Manufacturers = Hide

Would you trust your spouse it he or she was hiding things? Likewise then, you wouldn't trust a food company that does the same, and refuses to answer or provide information about the product's ingredients.

Now the cover says, No MSG "Added". This means what? Well, they didn't "add" any MSG. But, is there MSG in it? Well that's possible. There are so many ways to get around this, and bad companies, companies that want to make you addicted to the product, so that you buy it every week, these "bad" companies know all the tricks to labeling. Use a different chemical, use di-sodium glutamate, or mono-potassium glutamate, just modify the chemical slightly and now you can say "No MSG".

So this is where we go internally for guidance. And I will say that this product has a bit of a "hook" to it. Just like the TJs barbecue sauce said it had "kick". But this recipe formula dilutes out the "kick" by adding rice, additional chicken, and hempseed. I only make this recipe once a year, so clearly I am not going back to the store every week to purchase it because I'm "hooked" on it.

Nutrition Facts
5oz 140g servings about 4
E=260
F=70
Na=500
CHO=35g
Prot=13g
Try to find one that matches this. We will be using 1/4th of the box per serving, 624g÷4–156g, 156g/140g–1.11, so we multiply our label by 1.114, E=290 F=78 Na=557 CHO=156 f=0 s=62 Prot=58 T=292, 53 27 20.

2. Organic Basmati Rice
TJs brand, 32oz 907g, $3.99, organic white basmati rice. We will use 240g for the recipe, about a quarter of the bag. This is a stock item. I store the remainder in a 32oz glass sks jar with screw cap. Recall that the screw cap creates an airtight seal for best storage.

The nutrition facts say 50g E=180 F=0 CHO=39g Prot=4g. We will have 15 (uncooked) grams per serving, E=54 F=0 Na=0 CHO=47 f=0 s=0 Prot=5 T=52, 90 0 10. If your rice has 5 calories of fat, F=5, it will be fine.

The fiber is zero, it's white rice. Brown rice has fiber. But the white rice goes better with this recipe, and we will have brown rice in the NCD Chicken Bowl™, so to make things interesting, we have white rice here, and in the NCD Curry Chicken™. You eat it and then it's out of your system. You don't feel deprived.

3. Chicken Breast – boiled, same as before
You will add 2.1oz cooked chicken to each serving, x16=34oz total. How much is this of raw chicken? Divide by 0.75, 34oz÷0.75=45oz, divided by 16oz=2.8 pounds of raw chicken, plus some extra because you'll trim off a little fat, so, 3 pounds of raw chicken. Again, I usually buy the 6 lb value-pack and make BBQ Chx Peanut Butter Chocolate! You'll never get bored of that one!

pH
You are a pH expert by now, I hope. Otherwise this recipe book is going to be hard to understand. So if you haven't read the book, DO IT. Stop wasting your money on useless "stuff" and read the book so you can not only, "Take Control Of Your Weight By Taking Control Of The Numbers" but you will discover a key to health that is completely hidden in the mainstream – pH.

And it's true. You cannot see, touch, hear, or smell pH. It's the hidden aspect to our health that's completely overlooked when looking at root causes. Hence, root causes are not found, just treated.

Recall that our kidney beans softened when we added baking soda to the soak water. So when boiling your chicken, if the water is pH 5, your chicken will be a bit tough and hard to cut. If your water is pH 7.5 or higher, the chicken will be a bit soft, slightly mushy when you slice it. The ideal pH for boiling your chicken is 7, which is the textbook pH of pure water. So use the baking soda to adjust the water to pH 7, then write it down so you know how much you need when you make chicken again. Add 2 gallons of water to a 20L stockpot, remove a spoonful of water and test the pH with your 6-8 paper. If it's 7, then you're good-to-go. If it's less-than 7, then add a level tablespoon of baking soda, stir, and check it again. You don't need to use the potassium bicarbonate as it's more expensive, save that for your ABC Water™, just use the sodium bicarbonate baking soda that you bought from the baking aisle.

That whole-wheat spaghetti that we boiled for 30 minute in the roasted peppers chx pasta recipe, Chapter 13, that water was pH 5. You could probably shorten the time to 20-25 minutes if you use water with a pH of 7.

Do you see how pH affects things?

It's number one of my top-ten list for a reason.

Our 2.1oz cooked chicken breast is E=84 F=7 Na=53 Prot=73 T=80.

4. Organic Hempseed
Lassen's Healthfoods, Nutiva brand, 8oz 227g, $7.49, raw, shelled, refrigerate after opening, use within 12 weeks, nonGMO verified.

Okay, what do we know about hemp seeds? It's #3 in omega-3 fatty acid content. Flax Seeds Chia Seeds Hemp Seeds, Flax Chia Hemp. Then walnuts. Flaxseed is our "go-to" food for omega-3. Chia seeds are fine too, but why go with #2 when you can have #1.

Let's crunch our Hempseed.
3T 30g servings about 8
E=170
F=130
SF=1g low in saturated fat, just so you know
TF=0 no man-made fat, but you knew that
Polyunsaturated Fat = 11g x9 = 99 calories of omega 3 & 6

Monounsaturated Fat = 2g x9 = 18 calories of omega-9 OAP
(this is not an omega-9 food)
Chol=0 not found in plants
Na=0
CHO=2g x4 = 8 calories
f=1g x4 = 4 calories
s= <1g = "zero"
Prot=10g!! x4 = 40 calories
T=130+8+40=178
T-f=174
4.5 73 22.5
Macros with the fiber subtracted = 2 75 23

So I would say this food product is a fat, 73-75% fat, as we expect from seeds. It's very low carb, 2-4.5%, and high in protein, 23%. Nice.

Notice that our box of mandarin orange chicken was only 20% protein. The product says "chicken", but it's only 20% protein. These hemp seeds are seeds, fats, and are 23% protein. These seeds have more protein than the packaged chicken.

Nutiva says on their label, "Shelled hemp seeds contain 33% protein by weight." But we just said 23%. Well, this again is like our 96/4 ground beef that's 4% fat but it's really 33% fat when you crunch it.

Here's how they got the 33% protein. 10g of protein in a 30g serving, 10/30x100=33%. 33% protein by WEIGHT. But your body doesn't care about the "weight" of it. Your body only sees three things, carbs fats protein. And yes it sees vitamins, minerals, phytonutrients, etc., we covered all that in ABC NCD. The lesson here is, don't be fooled by 33% protein and 4% fat on the label. You've got to crunch the numbers to see what it really is.

This product lists poly- and mono-unsaturated fats. Why? Because it's an omega food, high in omega 3 & 6. Recall that we need to seek out omega-3, which we have done in the flaxseed shake, and that omega-6 is also essential, but not a seek-out fat. We need it, but we don't need to go looking for it. This product supplies a good amount of natural unrefined omega-6 from food, along with a fair amount of omega-3.

3T 30g has 7.5g of omega-6 and 3g of omega-3, that's 67.5 calories and 27 calories respectively. So our fat breakdown looks like this.
F=130cal
Omega-3 = 27cal
Omega-6 = 67.5cal
Omega-9 = 18cal
Saturated = 9cal

What are the percents of each?
27/130x100=21%
67.5/130x100=52%
18/130x100=14%
9/130x100=7%
The fat in hempseed is 21% omega-3, 52% omega-6, 14% omega-9, and 7% saturated, (along with 6% of unlisted fat).

Those are the percents with regard to the fat in hemp seeds. What are the percentages with regard to the whole hemp seeds?

Well, our T, total calories of the hempseed, carbs+fat+protein number, was 178. So,
27/178x100=15%
67.5/178x100=38%
18/178x100=10%
9/178x100=5%

Our hemp seeds are 15% omega-3, 38% omega-6, 10% omega-9, and 5% saturated fat.

Do you remember what flax seeds were? See page 9. Flaxseed is 31% omega-3. Hempseed is 15%. Half. And chia seeds are in the middle. Flax Chia Hemp. Omega-3. Your unstable U-shaped fatty acid chains that the body cannot make, so you have to eat them.

Fresh.

Freshly Ground.

The oils in plants don't get moldy so you can see that it's spoiled. They turn rancid. And you may not notice it, unless you smell it.

Rancid oil is right down there with burnt and man-made.

These hemp seeds are highest in omega 6, then 3, then 9, with a little bit of saturated. The label also lists 0.6g of GLA, gamma linolenic acid, borage, black current seed, and evening primrose oils (page 222). GLA is the precursor to the anti-inflammatory hormone PG1, similar to DHA and EPA in fish oil and PG3. Bottom line, these oils when consumed FRESH activate the hormones that fix and repair your body, keeping you looking HYA. And the bad oils, burnt, rancid, man-made, and refined omega-6, damage your body, triggering the bad hormones to be released, and then you feel tired, worn out, and just attribute it to aging.

You don't have to get old with JPM.

In fact, our mission is to get, and keep, you looking Half Your Age.

MINERALS!
It just doesn't stop with these hemp seeds. One 3T-30g serving has 50% or your RDV of magnesium, 15% of your RDV of iron, 25% of your RDV of zinc, and 50% for phosphorus. But as you recall, the two nutrients we don't worry about are phosphorus and chloride. We get plenty. Phosphorus is found abundantly in colas, meat, and all fertilized plant foods, and chloride is found in everything that gets washed or fed with municipal water.

So our NCD Orange Chicken meal will have 100mg of magnesium, and if you have two per day, you will have gotten half your daily magnesium requirement, just from the hemp seeds!

AND, since we see 50% mag, 25% zinc, and 15% iron, we can

assume many of our other minerals are there as well. Excellent!

As a final note, I want to clarify our OAP fats, our Olives/oil, Avocados/guacamole, Peanuts/butter, monounsaturated omega-9s.

Olive oil is 76% omega-9
Avocado is 70% omega-9
Peanuts are 47% omega-9
Cashews are 70%, almonds are 78%, and macadamias are 71%.
So if somebody reading my books has read *Fat That Heal Fats That Kill*, they may notice that peanuts are not HIGH in omega-9.

But peanuts contain our essential omega-6. Essential, but not really a seek-out fat. Peanuts are 29% omega-6, so this is a nice natural way to get omega-6 from unrefined raw food.

Our omega-6 foods that we eat on the NCD are:
1. fresh, canned, or frozen corn – no refined corn oil
2. fresh raw sunflower seeds – no refined sunflower oil
Also, buying them in the shells is the best way to eat them.
The other two ways are, freshly shelled, and sunflower seed butter.
3. Walnuts are 51% omega-6, and our 4th source of omega-3.
4. And peanuts are 29% raw natural unrefined omega-6.

The NCD has a recipe meal using walnut butter that you make in an Ultimate Chopper. So think about buying one if you don't already own one. It's the perfect kitchen appliance for making your own seed and nut butters.

So as you will see as you go along, the NCD has you eating fresh food sources of omega-6, not refined omega-6. Nuts are part of the "secret special" breakfasts, and you will love how I do this. And so peanuts and peanut butter, since they are technically legumes and not nuts, are grouped with the other two raw uncooked fats, olive oil and guacamole. Pick one a week, NCD Chicken Caesar Salad, NCD Chicken Bowl, NCD My Favorite Breakfast, Olives, Avocados, Peanuts, OAP.

CHAPTER 19

NCD Food Prep Rule™

Step 1 – the day before
Discard the four boxes that the orange chicken comes in, place the four bags of sauce and two of the bags of chicken in the refrigerator. Place the other two bags of chicken in the freezer, you will thaw them four days from now, as they have no preservatives.

Step 2 – the next day
Bring your 20L stockpot of 2 gallons of water, pH adjusted to 7, to a boil. Make your sliced-and-diced chicken breast.

Step 3
Add 240g of rice to a large glass bowl, add 1lb 5.6oz = 21.6oz of water pH 5. This acidic water, pH 5, will make your rice slightly firm and less soft and mushy. I like my pasta soft and mushy and my rice firm-ish al dente. Swirl the bowl a little to even out the rice on the bottom of the bowl and microwave it 15 minutes.

Step 4
Open the bag of hempseed and transfer the entire contents to a 16oz sks jar with screw cap. You want them to stay fresh as they were removed from their shells at the factory, and so the clock is ticking on those unstable omega-3s.

Step 5
Place 16, 16oz sks jars on the counter and remove their lids. Add

one-fourth of the packet of mandarin sauce to each jar, 4 jars per packet. In the beginning you can weigh it. Place the jar on the scale, add 1.6oz 45g of sauce, repeat repeat repeat. Repeat with the other three packets of sauce. When you are done you will have 16 jars with sauce on the bottom.

Step 6
The bags of breaded chicken contain about 454g 16oz each, so each bag divides into four 4oz servings. Place the jar with sauce on the scale, zero it, add 4.0oz of the breaded chicken, repeat repeat repeat. Repeat with the second bag. You now have 8 jars with sauce and chicken and 8 jars with just the sauce.

Step 7a
Add 2.1oz of your sliced-and-diced cooked chicken breast to each of the 16 jars.

Step 7b
Tidy up some. Wash dishes and put them away, discard bags, etc.

NCD Food Prep Rule™

CLEAN AS YOU GO
Clean up as you go along, utilizing your one-minute here and your two-minutes there, so that when you are done making the recipe, you only have a couple minutes of cleanup to do and you can sit down and eat in a relaxed, peaceful, cleaned-up environment. ☺

Step 8
Your 15 minutes are up, and your rice is done. Remove it from the microwave and let it evaporate some, ~2 minutes. Your 240g of dry rice is now 625g of cooked rice, divided by 16 = 39g. Use a soupspoon to add 39g of cooked rice to each of the 16 jars. Use a scale in the beginning so that you know what 39g of cooked rice looks like. Then later on, you can omit the scale step to save time. Or, you can do the first jar using the scale, and now you have a visual reference of 39g. Then you can aliquot the remaining rice to the remaining 15 jars visually without using the scale.

Step 9 – final step
Cap all your 16 jars. Shake to Mix. Refrigerate. You will have 8
jars with everything, and 8 jars with everything except the breaded
chicken. After you've eaten 6 of your 16 meals, take the other two
bags of chicken from the freezer and aliquot them into the 8 jars
for meals 9-16.

Time to Eat!

Remove the cap and place your jar of mandarin-chicken-rice in the
microwave. Micro 1min for warm, add another 30sec for hot. You
can cover it with a paper towel, but I've never had it splatter.

Place the jar on the scale and add 14 grams of hempseed. Enjoy!
Hempseed, 227g÷16=14.2g E=80 F=61 CHO=4 f=2 Prot=19.

This tastes just like orange chicken you would get at a restaurant,
but it's WAY better for you. 30% protein, minerals, good fats,
fresh fats, and the carbs are there to make it taste good. There's no
vegetable, so be sure to have snap peas later on at your desk. Or
boiled green beans on the side. See Chapters 50-54 in the main
book for the complete NCD Free Vegetable Protocols™.

Our final numbers are:
6 16 32 44 54, and the powerball number is…☺
E=290+54+84+80=508
F=78+7+61=146
Na=557+53=610 You can expect 2-3x this at a fastfood outlet.
CHO=156+47+4=207
f=2
s=62
Prot=58+5+73+19=155
T=508
40.7% carbs, 28.7% fat, 30.5% protein, 41 29 30. As you can see
there's no significant fiber so we are not going to crunch it further.
There's a photo, with green beans, on the website, so check it out.
Cost per meal is $4.99x4 + $3.99x0.26 + $1.99x3lbs + $7.49 =
$34.48 ÷ 16 = $2.15, for this fun, healthy, macro-balanced meal!

CHAPTER 20

NCD Salmon MV Focaccia™

Okay! Time for some DHA and EPA!

I hope you are beginning to see that you are looking at food differently.

It's not so much what it looks like, IT'S WHAT'S IN IT.™

But with the NCD, I think you get both. It looks good and it's loaded with what your Divine Intelligence needs.

Recall that you can serve any of these on a plate. For the Orange Chicken, you can heat it, pour it onto a plate, sprinkle it with the 14g hempseed, then place a 4oz serving of cooked green beans next to it. Beautiful.

So for our Salmon Mixed Vegetables & Focaccia, we need 3 items and 5 items total.

1. canned red salmon
2. frozen mixed vegetables
3. focaccia bread

1. Red Salmon
TJs brand, wild caught, 7.5oz 212g, $3.99, x2 cans, pacific red salmon, salt, product of the USA – ALASKA!

1/4th cup 63g servings about 3.5
E=110cal
F=60cal
Prot=13g

Try to find one that matches this. We will be using half a can per serving, 212g÷2=106g÷63g=1.68, so we multiply our NF, nutrition facts, by 1.68. E=185 F=101 Na=454 Prot=87 T=188, 0 54 46. This salmon is almost 50/50 fat and protein. It's 54% fat and 46% protein. It's a fatty fish. And it's this fat in this fish that has our essential DHA and EPA.

2. Organic Mixed Vegetables – 2 lbs, 907g

TJs brand, Organic Foursome, 16oz 454g, freezer aisle, organic cut green beans, organic peas, organic carrots, organic corn, $1.69 each, buy two.

All NF for mixed vegetable are about the same, 85g = 50 calories. We will be using 8oz 227g, half the bag per serving, so 227g is E=134 F=0 Na=53 CHO=118 f=32 s=32 Pro=21 T=139, 85 0 15.

This bag of carrots, green beans, corn, and peas, is 15% protein. This is why vegans and vegetarians say you can get all the protein you need from plants. It's true. Unless you work out. If you don't work out, 15% protein is fine, to keep you alive. But what is happening to the person who is working out? That muscle soreness that you experience the next day is your body tearing down and rebuilding your muscles bigger and stronger to cope with the new challenge you gave it. This is MUSCLE TURNOVER.

The person who is not working out isn't having muscle turnover. Very little anyway. Now the weightlifter, whose workout is all about CHALLENGING AND WORKING YOUR MUSCLES, is going to be experiencing a lot of soreness the next day and therefore A LOT of muscle turnover. This person needs protein.

The 40%-protein bodybuilder meals are appropriate and needed for someone who has just completed a heavy intense weightlifting workout. An 8oz chicken breast would give your body 208 calories of protein, or 52 grams of protein. Two hours later, have another one. If you work your muscles fully and with a lot of focus on the muscle and on your form, your Divine Intelligence will be yelling "CHICKEN!" "I need chicken in here!", after your workout is over.

The point is, there is no one-size-fits-all.

The person who gets up, goes to work, sits at a computer, comes home, makes dinner, does the laundry, makes the lunches, and goes to bed, is active, but not turning over their muscle tissue.

This person can get by on 15% protein. But careful. Where is that other 15% going to go? Assume this person was eating 30% protein and decided to drop it to 15%. Well, most likely the person will eat more carbs. So they would be eating 55% carbs 30% fat 15% protein. The recommended protein amount on nutrition facts labels is 10%, along with the standard 30% fat and 60% carbs. But what do you see?

60% carbs + 30% fat with a little protein is CarbFats. Desserts.

This person had better watch their calorie intake because if you don't burn it off you will be storing it. And they had better not be eating these carbfat meals in the evening before bed.

If you did decide to eat this way, you would have to do 3 things.
1. Drop your caloric intake.
2. Track your calories thoroughly.
3. No eating 3-4 hours before bed. Kitchen closed at 6.

It's better to have extra protein in your diet than not enough. If you don't have enough protein, then you're short on protein and your body starts to malfunction, in small ways in the beginning and then in bigger ways as time moves on. However, if you don't have enough carbs, your body grabs some of the extra protein and makes energy from the protein. Not a problem for your body.

Fats and Proteins can function as Carbs, but Carbs cannot do what

Fats and Proteins can do.

So if you are going to be deficient in something, don't let it be proteins or essential fats. NCD Dietary Essentials™ page 223.

3. Tomato & Olive Focaccia Bread
This is so yummy! Since you are being good by eating salmon and vegetables, you get to be bad by having this white-flour cheese bread. TJs brand, 15oz 425g $3.49, buy one. Enriched unbleached flour (wheat flour, malted barley, niacin, iron, thiamine mononitrate, riboflavin, folic acid), provolone cheese (cultured milk, enzymes, salt), mozzarella (cultured pasteurized part skim milk, enzymes, salt), diced tomatoes (tomatoes, tomato juice, salt, citric acid, calcium chloride), green olives, onions, canola oil, parmesan cheese (pasteurized cultured milk, enzymes, salt), garlic, basil, oregano, rosemary, thyme, crushed red pepper, yeast, salt.

Are they hiding anything? Nope. If you called this company and asked them specific questions about their ingredients they would likely be very helpful and forthright. They listed all the spices that they use, by name. Nice.

It's a long list of ingredients, but it's really just white bread and cheese with an onion-olives-spices topping. Simple. You could make it yourself.   But why bother when this is essentially homemade.

2oz 56g servings about 8
E=120
F=20
CHO=20g
Prot=5g
Try to find one that matches this. You will be dividing it into 4, so 425÷4=106g. When it comes to bread products, weigh them to be sure it really is what it says it is. The actual weight of this was 436g, 11g higher, so we will be getting 3g additional per serving, or, 109g instead of 106g. It's not worth taking into consideration in this case. So, 106g/56g=1.89, we multiply our NF by 1.89.

E=228 F=38 Na=512 CHO=152 f=0 s=0 Prot=38 T=228, 67 17 17. If you are crunching along with me, you may be getting slightly different numbers, i.e., 120x1.89=227. For best accuracy, you should crunch all-at-once, and then round off at the end. For example, 425g÷4÷56gx120cal=227.6=228.

This focaccia is 67% carbs, 17% fat, 17% protein. Now just suppose you were going to eat a diet of 70% carbs 15% fat 15% protein. You would basically be eating this cheese bread for all of your meals. Not only would you risk becoming visibly fat, but you would be missing out on all the other great foods. People that eat this way generally don't work out, or if they do, they do LBC, long boring cardio. You know, the people at the gym lined up on the elliptical machines with their Walkman and earbuds. These people are intent on burning off calories, because they are eating 60-70-80% carbs! Even if they don't have visible body fat, their bodies still look fat because their muscles are soft and laced with fat from their excessive carb intake.

High carb is for the INTENSE exerciser. The Anaerobic exerciser.

The anaerobic-exercise person is burning calories at a rate 18-times higher than the aerobic-exercise person. Hence, the name LONG and boring, versus, short and INTENSE. Many "experts" will advise against intense anaerobic exercise, claiming that it is too strenuous on the body. They say, intense exercise is too intense for your body, that the body wasn't designed for intense exercise. Well, if you want to believe that, then go ahead and baby your body, and stick to doing LBC workouts. You can reward yourself with a jar of pablum after your workout is over. The take-home message is, Be Sure To Include Intense Exercise into your routine, and especially if you want to burn calories.

Sadly, there are thousands of people who fit this profile, high-carb diets and long boring cardio. They would do themselves more benefit by skipping the gym and reading this book.

CHAPTER 21

Masterpiece

Thaw the mixed vegetables in the refrigerator overnight, or two hours at room temperature.

Step 1
Add the two cans of salmon to a large flat-bottom bowl, include the liquid as well. Using the back of a steak knife, peel off the skin and discard it, breaking up the salmon as you do so. Be sure to leave the bones in the bowl, that's your calcium for the day.

Step 2
Using a potato masher, mash the salmon and bones and mix it around with the liquid until it becomes a homogeneous bowl of salmon.

Step 3
Add your 2 bags 2 lbs of mixed vegetables to the salmon. This TJs brand of frozen vegetables doesn't need to be drained as there's no water, but if you buy a different brand, hold the opening of the bag and invert it over the sink to drain off any water.

Step 4
Mix your salmon vegetables. Aliquot it into four 16oz sks jars with the screw caps, filling each jar to the very top, completely 100% full. It divides up perfectly into these four 16oz jars. The weight of the batch is 1286g÷4=321g each. But you don't need to

use the scale. Just fill each jar to the top, full, pat it down some if you need to make it fit. Cap & Refrigerate.

Step 5

Open the plastic of the focaccia and cut it into 4, top to bottom, left to right, TBLR. This product has a thin-cardboard bottom so we are using that as the "cutting board" and so less dishes to wash. This focaccia is an 8-inch by 8-inch square, so when you are done cutting it, you will have four 4x4-inch squares. Now, cut each 4x4 square into cubes and stuff the cubes into a 16oz sks jar and cap it. They fit perfectly as well. And this way, you don't have to worry about spoilage because it's airtight. Repeat with the other three 4x4 squares, cutting each 4x4 into cubes and placing the cubes into the 16oz jar and capping it. Refrigerate them.

If you want to weigh your 4x4 squares to be sure they are all equal, they should be 106g each, or in this case, 3g more, 109g.

You now have four meals. Place the 16oz jar of focaccia bread on top of the 16oz jar of salmon-vegetables. They look so nice stacked like this, and then you just grab the two jars and sit down with a fork. Option – the medium pyrex rectangle also works.

If you want to eat from a plate, just empty the salmon-vegetables onto a plate, and then place the cubes of focaccia next to it. Beautiful. See the website for a picture of it.

This can also easily be taken "to go" and eaten at work, in your car, or at a picnic table at the park.

E=185+134+228=547
F=101+38=139
Na=454+53+512=1019 1 gram of sodium is fine
CHO=118+152=270 net carbs=238
f=32
s=32
Prot=87+21+38=146
T=555

T-f=523

Macros = 49 25 26

Macros with fiber subtracted = 45 27 28

If you check my calculations, which I hope you have been doing so you get the hang of it, you will see that the 45 is really 45.5 and I rounded it down so that we wouldn't end up with 101%, 46+27+28=101, whereas 45+27+28=100. The fat was 26.6, so it got rounded up to 27, if we round up twice, we end up with 101.

This looks too high in carbs but it's not. There is 8oz of vegetables and so a lot of digestion is going to have to happen before the carbs in the vegetables get released. Half the carbs of this meal are the vegetables, and carrots and green beans are not usually counted, but because they are mixed-in with the corn and peas as one product, they got counted. Our mixed-vegetable CHO is 118 calories. Just suppose the starch vegetables, (peas and corn), make up 80 calories, and the carrots and green beans make up the remaining 38 calories. Then if you subtracted 38 carb calories, this meal would be pretty close to 40 30 30.

Also notice that there is very little sugar, 32 calories, and it's all vegetable sugar. So, the carbs being a little higher is just right. Any less and you'll be wanting dessert, coffee, or a soft drink to get you going afterwards.

Bottom line, the carbs in this meal are wrapped up and slow. There is no insulin spike.

Pros. So what are the pros and cons of this meal? I like to include a few just to remind me of why I am doing this. The pros are, salmon, 101 calories of fish fat per meal; color, yellow, green, and orange vegetables, and eight ounces of vegetables per meal; spices, garlic, rosemary, oregano, thyme, all spices are antioxidants; and 30% protein to sustain you. One minor con, price per serving is $3.71, slightly over the target, but no biggie.

I'm going to take a bow now if it's alright with you. This recipe is a masterpiece of nutrition, numbers, and fun!

CHAPTER 22

But there's more!

You're not done yet! We are going to do the variation of this recipe and substitute egg rolls for the focaccia, ah!

1. Chicken Egg Rolls
TJs brand, 4 egg rolls, 12oz 340g, $3.29, freezer aisle, buy two. Filling: skinless white chicken meat, chinese cabbage, bok choy, bamboo shoot, water chestnut, carrot, scallion, wheat flour, seasoning (salt, sugar, black pepper, garlic powder), sesame seed oil.

All foods right? Seasoning. Nice. See how they disclose what they are using for seasonings. Salt & Pepper, Sugar, Garlic Powder. Foods. This is a company you can trust. In fact, Trader Joe's is a supermarket you can generally trust. Food companies that say they are trying to protect their proprietary information are simply hiding the addictive food chemicals they are putting in their products. Vote them out $!

Crust: enriched flour (wheat flour, niacin, reduced iron, thiamine mononitrate, riboflavin, folic acid, enzymes), water, egg, salt, corn starch. Fried in canola oil.

Do you see how enriched white bread products is so bass-ackwards? You refine out the natural B vitamins and iron in the grain, then you fortify it back in using synthetic B vitamins and tainted iron metal. Apparently, someone took a strong magnet and held it over some iron-fortified cereal flakes and they were able to pull the cereal flakes up to the magnet. I never saw this as I never bothered to check into it further, as I am already AWARE of much of what goes on by certain evil food manufacturers. Read the ingredients on a soda pop and then look at the price and ask yourself where the value is for your money. Buy a one-liter bottle of cola at a minimart and see how much they are charging for it.

People get upset because they feel they can't do anything about the politicians in office. I understand that. BUT you do have spending power over your food. Your money-spending choices that you make every day determines what foods we have available for us to eat. Together, we could put all of them out of business in a year and have "homemade" food on our supermarket shelves and all organic produce and organic-fed beef, pork, and poultry.

Reality Check. Since that's not likely to happen anytime soon, you are going to have to make your own meals and search for companies that make "homemade" food.

So our egg rolls are "fried" in canola oil. This is likely to be deep fried at 425 degrees. Well, enjoy them. But you don't eat them every day. Rarely to Occasionally is fine.

The Nutrition Facts say,
1 egg roll 85g servings 4
E=140cal
F=25cal
Na=490mg
CHO=20g
Prot=8g
Try to find one that matches this, and be sure to get the chicken egg rolls so there's some protein, 8g.

We will be having two per meal! E=280 F=50 Na=980 CHO=160 f=8 s=16 Prot=64 T=274, 58 18 23. So these egg rolls are 23% protein, not bad, and they're not high in fat, only 18%.

Thaw them overnight in the refrigerator.

Step 1 – the next day
Place the packages of 8 egg rolls, 2 packs of 4, on a toaster-oven tray, or you can use your oven. I like my big toaster oven because it's quick to heat up, and then it doesn't heat up your entire kitchen like an oven can. I use the third position from the top for my egg rolls, and then place an empty tray in the top-rack position. Apparently those oven-heating elements are toxic and cancer causing, so you don't want to have them directly above your food. Turn it to 350° Bake, set a timer. At 10 minutes, use tongs to turn all the egg rolls over. Bake 10 more minutes.

If you thawed them overnight, then they will be cooked all the way through and taste just right. If you overcook them they will taste like crappy fastfood egg rolls. If you only thaw them on the counter for an hour and cook them 10 minutes and 10 minutes, they'll be doughy and undercooked – yuck. BUT, if you thaw them overnight, then cook them 10 minutes, turn, 10 minutes, they will be perfect, just right. Mmm!

Record your cooking times so that when you get it right you know what you did!

I was cooking with someone once and he made this awesome salad with sour cream, salsa, peanuts, avocado, romaine lettuce, chicken, and when he went to make it again later on, it wasn't even close to being the same. Too bad he didn't take notes. An amazing recipe, gone.

Step 2
Grab 4 of your medium glass pyrex rectangles with the red lids. I don't know what else to call them. They come in three sizes.
1. Small = 7x5x1.5 inches 750mL 3cups
2. Medium = 8x6x2 inches 1.5L 6cups
3. Large = 9⅜x7¼x2¾ inches 2.6L 2.75qts
It says "microwave safe" on the bottom of the glass. Apparently those plastic food containers that people used all these years

weren't safe to put in the microwave. Imagine that.

Buy 8 large, 8 medium, and 16 small, so that you have containers to put your meals in. They will last a lifetime. Mine still look new and they're ten years old, and I've never had one break or chip.

Have you replaced your Teflon pots and pans for ceramic yet?

Place the 4 medium rectangles on the counter and add 2 egg rolls to each. Then add your salmon-vegetables, 321g to each. Let the egg rolls cool, if they haven't already, and then cover and refrigerate.

Fresh out of the oven these egg rolls are delicious, and satisfies the desire for egg rolls. You can eat the remaining meals cold, or if you want you can remove the lid and microwave it 1min 30sec.

E=185+134+280=599
F=101+50=151
Na=454+53+980=1487   (you'll want 8oz of water later)
CHO=118+160=278   netCHO=238
f=32+8=40
s=32+16=48
Prot=87+21+64=172
T=188+139+274=601   T is also equal to 151+278+172=601
T-f=561
Macros = 46 25 29
Macros-f = 42 27 31
Cost=$4.49

Again, don't concern yourself with the 46 and 42% carbs just because it's not 40. Those are vegetable carbs and the sugar is low, plus the sugar is in the vegetables. So its glycemic load is perfect.

Also don't worry about the total calories of 601 and 561 as the vegetables contribute 139 calories. Eight ounces seems like a lot of vegetables, but if you use less, your salmon will taste too fishy. The vegetables dilute out the salmon flavor to…Just Right!

Certain doctors and PhDs who have written books tends to have a special area that they know more about than anyone else. For Dr. Clark is was pollutants and parasites, for Dr. Barry Sears it was the discovery that the optimum macros are 40% carbs 30% fat 30% protein, Dr. Erasmus's is dietary fats, Dr. Wallach, minerals, etc. For skin youthfulness the guru is Dr. Nicholas Perricone, *The Perricone Promise.* I got a chuckle out of his "dedication" on page 3. It says, "To my children" and it lists the names of his 3 kids. No mention of his wife, the Ex. Anyway, a certain rock star called him up asking for advice for his bad skin. Dr. Perricone sent him a case of canned salmon. It's a great book, the best advice for good skin.

If you've read ABC NCD then you know the preferred choice for salmon is canned.
1. it's protected from oxidation by light
2. it's protected from oxidation by air
3. it's wild, not farm raised

Be sure to become a JPM member for the third Salmon-MV variation with Steak Fries & Ketchup. It makes 16 and includes three squares of dark chocolate! And french fries every day!

Chapter Endnote
The dictionary lists the word "hmm" but not the word "hm". Technically, neither of these are words, they're just sounds. When you communicate with people in person, they will say, "hmm" long and other times "hm" short. So, JPM uses this also. Same goes for "mmm" and "mm", or even "mmmmmmm!" Clearly, they all have different levels of meaning.

Others that you will see are:
uh = hesitation
huh = upset, disappointment
ah = pleasure, or surprise, or realization
uh-oh = alarm
sooo = extremely
oooh = joking enthusiasm

CHAPTER 23

NCD Franks & Fruit™

So we were good by having the salmon and mixed vegetables, now let's be bad. Do you wanna be bad? Let's be bad.

Now I will admit that the name I gave this recipe is a bit lame, but, when choosing a name for a recipe, I consider what I like and what I don't like. "Chicken Tremendous" tells me only that the recipe has chicken in it. "Beef Magnifico", same thing. I like recipe names that spark my mind into telling me what it is. "Roasted Peppers Chicken Pasta", okay, there's roasted peppers, chicken, pasta, oh, that's the one with the sundried tomatoes, olive oil, and zucchini. Oh okay. So, sorry about the nerdy sound of this recipe title, but my goal is to make it so that when you see the "file titles" you know what's in the "file".

Do you ever create files on your computer and then later on you don't remember what's in those files? Same thing applies here.

So for franks and fruit you'll need 3 items, franks, fruit, and mustard. See, easy to picture it.

1. Extra Lean Beef Franks XXL
And they are XXL franks. Hoffy brand, Smart and Final, $4.99, 4g of fat per serving. This is different than 4% fat ground beef, which is 33% fat calories. This 4g of fat per frank is correct, 4x9=36cal, and the Fat Cals say 35. So when you see grams of fat, they are

talking nutrition facts, whereas percent fat is misleading in that it refers to fat by weight.

1 frank 90g, servings per container 10 (it's the Family Pack of 10)
E=90
F=35
CHO=5g
Prot=10g
Try to use the Hoffy brand or find one that matches the above. Buy one pack, it will aliquot into 5, two franks per serving. This recipe is a Snack, as the calories are 250, so it's a meal in the sense that it's 40 30 30, but it's a snack in terms of calories, 250.

Ingredients: beef, water, modified corn starch, contains less than 2% (uh-oh, here it comes), flavorings, paprika, extractives of paprika, corn syrup, soy sauce (soybeans, maltodextrin), salt, whey protein concentrate, hydrolyzed soy protein, dextrose, potassium lactate, sodium phosphate, sodium erythorbate, sodium diacetate, sodium nitrite, contains milk and soy. Recall our focaccia long list of ingredients and there was no "contains less than 2%" phrase. That phrase on a food label is a RED FLAG. Keep that in mind.

Well, the first ingredient is beef, so that's good. But it lists "modified" corn starch. Modified how? Why do you have to "modify" corn starch? Maltodextrin, which is the same as modified or hyrdrolyzed corn starch, so why do we need both? Because maltodextrin has free glutamate for "kick". I am not going to go into all of this as it would take an encyclopedia to cover just the ingredients, thus, we have the three NCD basic rules.

NCD Ingredients Rules™
1. If it's not a food, it's a chemical, a chemical additive.
2. Rarely and Occasionally is fine, but not in moderation.
3. Your body is designed for toxin breakdown and removal.

You can explore these additives on your own, if you want. The NCD focuses on the GOOD things, the POSITIVES, we should be doing, while merely being informed and aware of the bad.

And I said we were going to be bad! If you talk to people about what they eat, you'll hear people say, "I just like to have a hot dog every so often." For me, this is true also. Once about every 12 months, I just like to have these franks. But it is more likely to be the yellow mustard seed that my body is asking for.

2. Yellow Mustard

Heinz brand, S&F $1.59, 17.5oz 496g, distilled white vinegar, water, mustard seed, mustard bran, salt, turmeric, paprika. But why not buy TJs organic mustard, organic grain vinegar, water, organic mustard seed, salt, organic sugar, organic turmeric, organic paprika, organic spices. Doesn't that sound better? There's no "hook" in this mustard so I will assume those spices are just spices, plus, since it says organic spices then isn't not likely to be Chemical Spices.

The calories are free, but we'll count the sodium. So two franks and the mustard look like this:

E=180
F=70
Na=1380+645=2025mg >1g and >2g!
CHO=40
f=0
s=8
Prot=80
T=190

That 645mg of sodium is from the mustard. I use $1/10^{th}$ of the heinz mustard bottle, so about 50g or 10t 3.3T. That's a lot, but yellow mustard-seed color is so good for you. When I have finished eating these five snack meals, I will have consumed the entire TJs container of organic yellow mustard, or half the heinz bottle. I am pretty sure this is the reason why I have this every so often, for the whatever-it-is that's in the yellow mustard seed.

I've never heard my inner Divine Intelligence say, "Hey, I need maltodextrin, we're out in here." "And throw in some modified corn starch and some hydrolyzed soy protein while you're at it."

Yeah, that just doesn't happen when it comes to body function.

3. Fruit – 75 net carb calories (fiber subtracted)
I am going to use 3oz of banana, or you could have, 6oz of apple, 7oz of apricot, 4.5oz blackberries, 7oz blueberries, 8oz cantaloupe, 5oz cherries, 4oz grapes, 7oz honeydew, 4.5oz kiwi, 4.5oz mango, 6.5oz nectarine, 6.5oz orange flesh, 7oz peach, 5oz pear, pineapple, or plums, 4.5oz pomegranate seeds/arils, 25g black raisins, 3.5oz raspberries, 11oz of strawberries, or 9oz of watermelon.

Now don't those choices sound good! This is why the NCD uses fruit for dessert, and in the recipes. We can not be excluding fruit from our diet. And we have to be careful when eating fruit because it's 100% sugar. Fine if you're active, less fine if you're not.

So the question becomes: How Then Do We Consume Fruit?

Well, this is how. For dessert. As a portion of the 200 calories of carbohydrate in our meal.

This way we can have our sugar, fruit, and not worry about gaining weight, as it's part of the meal.

You know, many people have lost fat simply by doing ONE thing.

They stopped drinking sodas (pop, soft drinks).

When you stop drinking soda pop, you stop consuming sugar. That bag of liquid dextrose IV solution that is being pumped into your veins gets turned off. Insulin goes down. And you stop storing any excess food that you consume as fat, but instead, you're burning it.

Go back and reread that paragraph. That paragraph is the reason for being overweight.

Or, if it's not sodas, it's lattes, or cookies, or some other sugar food that you are putting in your body as an added EXTRA. That IV bag of glucose/dextrose has lots of different names. Pretzels?

That list of fruit will be expanded on and summarized into a user-friendly chapter. Stay tuned for that! For now, let's get you started on the recipes and eating 40 30 30 macros with 500-calorie servings so you can get control of the numbers you're eating by tracking pre-counted meals.

So, putting the two together, we have Franks & Fruit,
E=180+0+75=255
F=70
Na=1380+645+0=2025
CHO=40+79=119
f=11
s=8+57=65
Prot=80+3=83
T=190+82=272
T-f=261
43.8 25.7 30.5 rounded = 44 26 30
Using T-f, 41.4 26.8 31.8 or 41 27 32 and $1.41 per serving.

Don't worry about exactness. We are TARGETING 40% carbs 30% fat 30% protein. The NCD stays within a reasonable range. AND, we are also LISTENING to our divine intelligence for how the meal feels, because food labels are not 100% accurate anyway.

Some of the recipes come out exactly 40 30 30 on paper, but that doesn't mean to say it will FEEL 40 30 30. We keep the carbs at 40 41 42 or 43% with 44 being the high side and 45 being the limit.   The Salmon-MV meal, again, half of those carbs were vegetable carbs. As the carbs go up, then the fat or protein or both will come down, as they all equal 100%. So protein is the key one. We don't want to let our protein drop too far below 30%. Otherwise what? What? Dessert. Carbfats. Notice in this recipe the macros are 30% protein and with the fiber subtracted it's 32%. So we are keeping our protein steady.

Don't you love this!
Share this with a friend, and recommend my books to them. You'll see why they won't find the complete solutions, next.

CHAPTER 24

Hiatus

I should have also said in that last recipe that you can always use half the fruit amount and go Low Carb, or you can eliminate the fruit completely and go full atkins. It's up to you. The Number Crunch Diet is a flexible program. It works for all three goals, weight gain, weight loss, and weight maintenance. Because it's a Numbers-Based plan.

The NCD – a Mathematical Approach to Weight Management™

So this chapter does not have a recipe, but instead, we're going to work on your awareness. You can't change what you buy and how you eat until you stop to look at it.

The NCD is a holistic program, we look at the whole picture. In the *ABC Water and the Number Crunch Diet* we discussed parasites, yeast, chewing, praying, chlorine, plastics, and on and on. We even included spirituality, because...We Are Not Just Animals. We have a spiritual side. And that means a Creator. God, Jesus, Allah, whatever you prefer to call it, but you are more than just the Outer You. You're Two Yous. And the inner one is the Divine one, that just seems to know right from wrong, good from bad. You are free to pick your religion on the NCD, but we do believe in a Divine Creator God of some sort, and we look to this when making food choices, or any choices, and WHEN TRYING TO DISCERN THE TRUTH ABOUT THINGS.

If Jesus said the truth will make you free, then without it you are what? Not free. A slave. A prisoner. You are owned or controlled by others.

Where am I going with this you ask? The Media, mainstream.

NCD Foundational Principle™
If what you believe and know to be true is coming from the mainstream media, magazines, new headlines, television programs, "popular" books, you are in danger of being a slave or prisoner.

They simply aren't giving you the truth, which has to be the full truth or it's not "true", partial truths are technically not truths.

Here's what I mean.

Since I shop at Smart and Final, they send me a mini magazine for restaurant owners. Here's what they have to say in this month's issue.

"One of the reasons for the 7.2% decline in diet soft drink sales is because of people's perception that they're not good for you."

OMG (oh my God). Are people that dumb. I was one of those people. Until you break free from the mainstream, you are that dumb. You're a slave. And you don't even know it.

Once you connect with your inner divine, you know INSTINCTIVELY what's good and what's not good, aka, evil, bad. And it happens in the snap of a finger, boom! INSTANTLY. Just like how a hypnotist snaps his finger to wake you up in an instant, your Divine Intelligence goes off Instantly.

As you begin to connect with your inner intelligence, the "instantly" can become 2-3 seconds before the moment. Before something is about to happen, occur, or be said, you know two seconds before. You almost begin to operate from a place outside of current time. You are becoming less external. Less outer world.

The more and the closer you can connect to that Divine Intelligence, the more you will see what's really going on around you. DISCERNMENT

Oh, I love that word. But the mainstream rarely uses it. Why? Because they don't want you to Discern. If you discern what they are feeding you, you will see right through it, and you will see it for what it really is. UNTRUTH.

JPM UNtruths™
1. Partials – they tell you part of the story, but not the whole story.

2. Clouded – they tell you some truth, but it's so discombobulated you can't make sense of it, so you just say, ok, and go along with it.

I worked with a woman and she would go on-and-on-and-on about why this and this was not done. I had to really pay close attention to what she was saying so I could DISCERN the truth. The truth was, she was lying, and covering up the reasons for not getting it done. And her modus operandi was to just talk a lot and hopefully the other person wouldn't question it, or they'll just find it too exhausting to listen. Women are notorious for this. Ladies, no, ladies are noble. Women, and females, and effeminate men, in that order, are the worst for doing this. Recognize it and Discern it.

3. Partial Plus – this is where they tell you some truth but not the whole truth, then they throw in some lies. "SPIN" – they spin it. They say something true to give themselves credibility, then they lie, then they throw it back at you. Anyone can play this game. Except noble men and women. They will see it. AND they should counter it, when appropriate. I don't know about the God you work for, but the God I work for expects me to take a stand and speak up when appropriate and counter this spin with the truth.

4. No Truth – lies. People that just outright lie. Either they believe it to be true and dish it out as advice, or they know that it's not true and they dish it out as advice. As your discerning skills get better, you will be able to tell the two apart. You will be able to tell

if they, 1) believe the lies they are proclaiming, or 2) they know what they are saying is untrue but they are trying to sell you on it. So,

4a = they themselves are brainwashed and want you to be too

4b = they know darn-well, but they want YOU to buy into it

An example of 4a is the person who's been listening to a radio talk-show host, and armed with his 30 minutes of one-sided commentary, goes out into the world and tries to persuade everyone he meets that XYZ is bad, or good.

An example of 4b is the used-car salesman that tells you the car had one owner when in reality it's been bought and sold five times. We are all guilty of this, myself included. I've walked into the ER to draw blood on a patient, and there is a long list of orders on someone who says she has a headache. Then, back at the lab, I'd run all those tests and report them out. Everything was pretty much normal, nothing significant. $350 please. It's called, unnecessary workup. But that's only half of it. The other half is, to generate billing. If the doctor doesn't do it, the hospital fires him and gets someone that will. Welcome to the world.

So it's 2014 and the general public has just started to perceive that diet soft drinks aren't good for you.

Boy, do we have a long way to go.

Surely, if you've read ABC NCD and this book up to this point, you can see how JPM is going to have you MILES ahead of the average person. That's my job. To get you there. And to keep you there.

The next thing this magazine article says is, "There are questions about the health of sweeteners and sodium content." Well, I am not concerned about the "health" of sweeteners, but I am concerned about the health "consequences". See how they word it? THEY, the mainstream media, feeding you what to believe, so they can control you, and keep you a slave/consumer of their industry, they, don't want you to think about the CONSEQUENCES of your choices. That would mean listening to your Divine Intelligence for understanding. Instead of listening to them.

Also notice how they refer to the artificial sweetener in the diet drink as a "sweetener". Wrong. Sweeteners are thought of by most people as honey, sugar, maple syrup, and fruit juice. NutraSweet, Equal, and Splenda, are referred to as artificial sweeteners. Or more accurately, Chemical Sweeteners. So this article is trying to group them all together, honey maple syrup aspartame sugar sucralose fruit juice. It's subtle how they do this, but if you're not aware of it, then, over time, you'll come to believe they're all the same – they're all just sweeteners.

Then it says "sodium content", "People are concerned about the sodium content in soda pop." On page 109 of the main book, you will recall how people in the medical profession are told this as well. I once had a Physician's Assistant warn me about the sodium in pepsi. It's Phosphates that we need to be concerned about.

Colas are loaded with Phosphates.™
Teas are loaded with Oxalates.™

So pick your poison, you lose calcium either way. And to make matters worse, you just consumed calories with NO nutrition. Oh, that's right, that's why we switched to drinking diet.

If you follow what everyone else is doing, the mainstream followers, you will find yourself going around in a circle.

Break out of the mainstream and tell a friend about Jumper Publications – insider information for the elite thinkers.

The bulk of the populace will always be lost. And they'll lose everything in the end. This is another reason for the price of this book being significantly higher than most books.

Take the book *South Beach Diet* by Dr. Agatston. Hm, I just noticed our last names share a "g" and a "ston" and start with a vowel. Awareness – it will carry over into other things.

So this book is a New York Times bestseller. I was sold, I bought it. But that was in the beginning of my learning stages. And thank you to Dr. Agatston for his book, as I did learn from it at the time. But I've gone miles beyond that now. This #1 NY Times bestselling book is only 105 pages. What! It's a 310 page book, but 205 pages of it is the meal plan and recipes, blah blah blah. I call this filler. Some people do this with the index, or endnotes. Add 30-40 pages of index and endnotes to pad the book. Your publisher wants 300 pages but you've run out of advice and tips at 150. Or in this case, the advice and tips stop on page 106. How lame. And a number one bestseller. You could take any 60 pages in the *ABC Water and the Number Crunch Diet* and get just as much information as this 300-page NY Times bestselling book. Five to one. JPM books cost more because their 5 to 1 when it comes to tips, advice, and content.

And, more importantly, the JPM tips and strategies are coming from a do-it-yourself selfcare common-sense angle, not, a hand-yourself-over-to-a-profit-and-money-system/medical-system angle.

Lastly, this S&F magazine article says that, "People are shifting away to other beverages such as iced tea because the perception is that they are better for you." Well, they're not. And there you have your CIRCLE.

Chapter Endnote
JPM's "summary index" reads like a long chapter, a full-book review. It restates things for the purpose of solidifying the contents of the book. It is meant to be "useful", not "filler".

Prescient – having knowledge of an event before it takes place. Imagine being in this state every minute of every day, page 120-1.

CHAPTER 25

NCD Franks & Relish™

Okay, we're not done being bad! We have the variation.

Instead of 75 calories of fruit, we are going to have 75 calories of "relish", but not store-bought relish, we are going to make it ourselves from bread-and-butter pickles.

1. TJs Organic Sweet Bread & Butter Pickles, $3.49
The jar of pickles says it's 24 net fluid ounces, 710 mL. The pickles with liquid weigh 765g, and the pickles alone weigh 454g. So, you get 16 ounces of pickles in a 24oz jar of pickles. Yes, only an obsessive-compulsive person would figure that out.

If we aliquot the pickles/relish into 8, then our carbs are 65 calories per serving. There's no fiber, so let's go with 8 and 65. If you double this recipe and buy two packs of franks, you can have this snack every day for the next 10 days. Then for the 9th and 10th servings, have it with fruit, 25 grams of raisins works good. So, snacks 1-8 with the relish and snacks 9&10 with the raisins. You will have no urges for a hot dog after that. If you purchase just one 10-pack of franks and make 5 servings, then you can use the leftover relish as part of a meal, or you can eat a spoonful for free between meals, as it is a cucumber, (with a little added sugar).

The ingredients say, organic cucumbers, organic crystalized cane juice, water, organic distilled vinegar, salt, calcium chloride, organic dehydrated onions, organic dehydrated peppers, organic celery seed, organic mustard seed. Fantastic.

Organic Organic Organic, don't you love the sound of that word? The word itself says "wholesome, natural, healthy, and pure". Contrast that with the scary words on regular supermarket items like maltodextrin and modified blah-blah-blahs. Pickles are where you MUST read the label. The NCD says NO colors or dyes. All regular-brand pickles and pickle relish have YELLOW number, well the numbers vary. The point is, we only eat YELLOW phytonutrients, P. 229, not yellow dyes. That goes for blues and reds as well, red #40 blue #1 yellow #5&6, no dyes period.

Transfer the jar of pickles to a colander and then add the pickles to a food processer and chop 'em up. Pickle Relish! Tastes as good if not better and you'll never go back to using store-bought relish.

Transfer the relish to a 16oz sks jar with screw cap to keep it nice and fresh, or you can use a pyrex bowl with the red lid but it will dry out a bit as the days go by. The relish that doesn't fit in the 16oz jar is what you will use for your first serving.

The Hot Dog Express

No this is not a train, it's a wiener grill, the kind you see when you walk into a 7-Eleven. $50 and it's sooo worth it. Place your franks/wieners on the rollers, close the lid, and turn it to 30 minutes. The rollers turn the wieners and cook them evenly to perfection, mm! I cook 4 at a time, then I have 2 for my snack and leave the other 2 on the grill for a snack later on. So, it becomes a 500-calorie meal in two parts. That's why you won't see a lot of these 250-calorie snack recipes, because if you want a snack, you just have half a meal, half the Hawaiian Pizza for example.

If you are a man and work out, don't bother with 250-calorie snacks, as your caloric intake is 2500-3500-4000 a day. If you eat snacks, that would be 10-14-16 feedings per day. Not practical. You have time to eat 5-6-7 times a day, so stick with 500-calorie meals only. Or you can do 3 double meals of 1000cal each = 3000 per day, or 2 doubles and a single = 2500 calories, or 3 doubles and a single, 3500 calories. The NCD Orange Shake™ or the NCD Chocolate Milk™ work great for double meals. You have a solid-food meal along with your orange shake = 1000 calories. You can also do the double meal with the Flaxseed Shake, maple, honey, or molasses. The molasses shake might slow you down a bit because it doesn't have the sugar punch that maple syrup and honey have. And if you are going to eat 1000 calories, you are going to need more sugar to keep the brain happy while the body diverts blood glucose to your digestive system. If the glycemic load is too low, you'll not get the energy from the meal that you're supposed to. And that's the whole point right? Energy.

It seems in today's society, everyone wants more energy. "How do I keep from getting tired?" "I need more energy." "Not now, I'll do it later." And on and on and on. Well, if these people would just pay attention to their calories, and where they are coming from, they wouldn't have energy problems like they do.

E=XXX calories, that E that we've been referring to is ENERGY!

Then we double-check our E by calculating T.

T=XXX+XXX+XXX=XXX calories.   These numbers are calculated from our MACROS, Fat+Carbs+Protein.

Calories and Macros. Get those right and your energy will be there. If this is impacting you right now, buy a copy of this book for a friend or a relative.

So when your franks are ready, place them on a plate, place the plate on your scale, spoon on 56 grams of relish, and Enjoy. You can add mustard or mustard-and-onion for free. It becomes a hot dog with no bun. But who needs a white bun with enriched white flour? Your DI doesn't.

Not to worry because the NCD has full hot-dog recipes with the bun, NCD Chili Dog™ with kidney-bean chili, cheddar, and onions on a white hot-dog bun, and NCD Hot Dogs™, two hot dogs with mustard and a little chopped onion on white hot-dog buns, and 15 grams of CHOCOLATE. I've got you covered.

Seriously. After a while, you've had so much fun eating that you are bored with food. It's just not on your mind. It becomes, just food. And, you don't have food cravings, just an occasional urge or desire for something, because your body is stocked up with nutrients. The shelves in your pantry, (cells and tissues), are full.

For the Franks & Fruit version with the mustard, place the plate on the scale and add 50 grams of mustard. This will be a lot of mustard, but again, it's the mustard seed that your body wants. Your taste buds will be saying, "mmm that tangy mustardy flavor, that's what I was looking for", not "mmm maltodextrin".

Another shout-out to the Heinz Corporation. Recall that in the main book we praised Heinz over French's because Heinz stopped using "Natural Flavoring" in its yellow mustard. Well, someone at Heinz is really thinking because they came up with a new container design where the cap is on the bottom. This is what America is all about! People thinking outside of the box. Innovation! Creativity! So not only is there no air when you squirt it, but there's also no mess as it doesn't drip. You squeeze it and the mustard comes out, then, because it's under pressure now, when you release your hand, the mustard goes up inside the container and the spout stays perfectly clean. Amazing! The inventor of this is a genius. Not only is your mustard ready-to-squirt because it's upside down, but then the pressure keeps the spout clean so you never have to wipe it. Don't you love this great country of ours! Rather than "never forget this or that" campaigns, I say, never forget INNOVATION.

Our final numbers for this Franks & Relish are essentially the same as the Franks & Fruit, just a little less sodium without the mustard, but still over one gram. Just be aware that you'll want a glass of water a half hour later. No biggie. After all, we did say we were going to be bad!

CHAPTER 26

NCD Taco Salad™

There is one other thing I want to mention in that Smart and Final Business Advantage magazine for restaurant owners. And that is this, it goes on to say that lattes are very popular and big sellers because of the Starbucks craze. It says, "You can charge $3.50 a cup but it only costs 25-30 cents to make, that's a nice margin."

See. They are focused on margins, and profit, not on value for your money, or nutrition. Contrast this with our Trader Joe's reduced-sugar organic blueberry jam. Since they have cut back on the sugar, then they have to use double the blueberries, and organic blueberries. And they are packaging your food in nontoxic glass, more costly than plastic, and heavier to ship. But they care about their customers. This company is sacrificing profit to give you good food. Their profit margin may be as little as 10% by the time the supermarket takes their cut of your money.

The latte company is making 90% profit, and using YOUR money to pay for their luxury home in Maui, while giving you 25 cent of coffee, milk, and sugar. Your body gets nothing in return. Your money is as good as thrown in the trash.

VOTE better please.
Discern.

Make it TRENDY! Imagine how out-of-the-box cool you'll be

when your friend says, "Let's grab a coffee", and you reply, "Oh, I don't waste my money on that, it's 90% profit margins, and I get no nutrition in exchange." Imagine Saying That. Really. Do It!

Young people, you all want to express yourselves and be different with your tattoos and piercings and all that. I challenge you, be different with your thinking – think Out-Of-The-Box to be unique!

People in Los Angeles and New York are always looking to outshine and stand out from the others, well, think outside the box!

You'll need 8 different items and ~14 total items.

1. romaine
2. corn chips
3. cheddar
4. tomatoes
5. kidney beans
6. black beans
7. ground beef
8. taco seasoning

Think of it in 4 parts or layers, from the bottom up we have, romaine, chips, chili, cheddar.

1. Romaine Lettuce
FRESH!! Romaine Heads, 4 nice and green heads. Don't buy the romaine in the bag, the three-in-bag pack, that's romaine HEARTS, with the dark leafy green removed. You are eating this meal for the dark leafy greens. Time to be good again. I buy mine at S&F for $0.99, or at Food Maxx. It's not organic, but it looks fresh, dark green, and healthy. If you pay attention when you go to wash it you may or may not see suds. Pesticides. Or, they washed it with some sort of detergent water at the farm. Switch to a different supermarket next time if you see suds.

2. Baked Blue Corn Tortilla Chips, Salted
TJs brand, 7oz 198g, "made with organic blue corn", $1.99, 2 bags.

Front label "bragging", No Preservatives No Artificial Colors or Flavors. Hm. I'm starting to think those things are really bad for me. Good thing I'm paying attention. Ingredients: organic blue corn, good, no GMO corn, expeller pressed oil (canola, safflower, or sunflower), bad, refined, and the canola's probably GMO, salt, lime. It's certified organic by QAI, quality assurance international, but it's not USDA organic because the oil and lime are not organic. So, it's good, but it could be better. The healthfood store likely has baked chips with organic oil, but not for $1.99.

1oz 28g servings per container 7
E=110
F=15
CHO=22g
Prot=3g
Try to find one that matches this. We will use 1/6th of the bag or 33g, E=130 F=18 Na=189 CHO=104 f=9 s=0 Prot=14 T=136. Your turn. Calculate the macros on your own.

Tick tock tick tock tick tock…tick tick tick tick tick…hurry… time's up.

104/136x100=76.4%   18/136x100=13.2%   14/136x100=10.3%. Our percent carb is 76.4, but if we round it down we will end up with 99%, which is okay, but let's round it up so that we get 100% total. So 77 13 10. That looks nicer, makes more sense to the brain. As an added bonus, these blue chips come from blue corn, and since it's organic, there are no pesticides or chemical fertilizers or genetically-modified DNA. So we can say we are getting a serving of blue plant color, phytonutrient group PBB.

3. Cheddar Cheese
TJs brand, I buy the raw milk cheddar cheese, for the raw proteins and better probiotics. Buy 12oz 0.75lbs, $5.49/lb=$4.10. We will be using 1oz 28g so the nutrition facts don't need to be adjusted. E=110 F=80 SF=6gx9=54 Na=170 CHO=0 Prot=28 T=108, 0 74 26. This is cheese, so 54/108x100=50%, 50% saturated fat. But our RDV limit is 25g 225cal, so 6g 54cal is only a quarter of our

daily limit. No CHO carbs means no fiber no sugar. They are subgroups of carbohydrate so that's why I denote them with lowercase f and s. And so that f is not confused with F.

Ingredients: Unpasteurized cow's milk, salt, microbial rennet, cheese cultures. This next part is interesting. "We segregate ingredients to avoid cross-contamination with allergens." Then it says, "Made on shared equipment with soy." So the standard allergy disclaimer that we so often see is, "Made on equipment shared with wheat, milk, and soy." So the gist of all that is, this cheese is made of milk on equipment shared with soy but not wheat.

4. Canned Diced Tomatoes
S&F First Street brand, one ginormous 6 pound 6 ounce can, 2.89 Kg, $2.85. Great savings. Tomatoes, tomato juice, salt, calcium chloride and citric acid. You don't need seasoned or designer tomatoes because we are going to be seasoning the chili ourselves, in which case the NF for plain canned tomatoes are all about the same, E=25 for a 1/2cup. We will be using $1/12^{th}$ of the can 241g, E=50 Na=756 CHO=32 f=8 s=24 Prot=8 T=40, 80 0 20. These tomatoes are 20% protein. The only problem is, I would have to eat 8 of these ginormous cans to get my daily protein calories, 2500calx30%=750cal÷8cals of prot=94÷12servings/can=7.8cans.

I did promise you you'd be a math expert after a while.
And that two years from now you would able to number-crunch design your own recipes!

And that you'd stop forgetting where you parked your car at the mall!

If you do this into your 80s you can forget about dementia.
You can't just look HYA, you've got to have a sharp mind too!

5. Light Red Kidney Beans
S&F First Street brand, 16oz 1lb 454g, 1 bag of dry beans, $1.49. One ingredient, light red kidney beans. We will be using half the

bag for this 12-meal recipe. Same for the black beans. This means, that I will make this recipe again next week, so 12 more equals 24 meals total. I'm fine with that many. I eat two per day so my 12 meals are gone in a week. Then I make it again the next week. It's so good and satisfying that I could probably keep having them beyond 24 meals, but I stop at 24 as it fits. Trust me, 12 won't seem like that many once you try this. You'll need 24 before you get bored. If you do want just 12, then omit the black beans, as the recipe calls for one 16oz bag of beans per 12 meals. I'm going to make 24, so I need 2 bags, one kidney one black.

The NF for $1/24^{th}$ of the bag is E=63 F=0 Na=0 CHO=47 f=12 s=2 Prot=17 T=64, 73 0 27. Dried beans have zero sodium, canned beans do not. 27% protein, almost like 2% milk but without the fat. Front label bragging says "high in fiber, good source of iron". What's the percent fiber? Check it. 12/64x100=18.75=19% fiber. When the nutrition facts have double-digit minerals, take notice of it. These beans have 15% of our RDA of iron per serving, calcium 4%, but God made cows for our dietary calcium. Soil is not a big source of calcium, but luckily we have cows and goats. They eat grass all day long and take the tiny bit of calcium in the grass and concentrate it multiple times into milk. Calcium is the most abundant mineral in your body. In fact – You Have More Calcium In Your Body Than All Of Your Other Minerals Combined.

Where would we be without cows.

6. Black Beans
S&F brand, 16oz 454g, 1 bag $1.39. One ingredient, black beans. That's about as close to food at its base form as you can get. "High in fiber and a good source of iron", 25% iron this time. We can assume zinc, copper, magnesium, and the trace minerals are there as well. Plus, black plant food, phytonutrients.

$1/24^{th}$ of the bag will be E=63 F=2 Na=0 CHO=47 f=19 s=2 Prot=16 T=65, 72 3 25. What's the percent fiber of this one? 19/65x100=29%. These black beans have 53% more fiber than the kidney beans. 29-19=10, 10÷19x100=53% more fiber.

All this information is on the label. But only the Number Crunch Diet is looking at it this deeply.

With knowledge comes power, will-power!

So if you hear someone say, "Oh, beans are high in fiber", you can reply, "Yes, and black beans are 29% fiber."

Or maybe your teenage son will search his smartphone to see if you're right, and when he does, he'll think, "Hm, I guess my mom's smarter than I thought."

7. Ground Beef 96/4 extra-lean ground beef, same as before 3.3oz E=108 F=33 Na=57 Prot=74 T=107. If you are making 12 taco salads, then you will need 2.5 lbs and have half-a-pound left over. This is another reason why I make it again next week, so for 24 meals you need 5 packs of ground beef. BUT, only buy 3 packs now and 2 packs a week from now. You will vacuum seal the remaining half-pound from pack #3 and use it next week.

Next week we will buy the 4 romaine heads, 2 bags of baked chips, 12oz of cheddar, the huge can of tomatoes, and the 2 packs of beef. Half the beans from the first week will be stored for the second week, so you won't have to prepare the beans, (one less step). Also, you can streamline this by buying 4 bags of chips, two 12oz cheddar, and 2 of the huge cans of tomatoes. So then next week you just have to pick up 4 romaine and 2 beef.

For those of you that are doing just 12 taco salads, cook the 3lbs of beef, pull off 1/6th of it, eyeball it, and you can squirt some ketchup on top with your leftover relish, and have 4 squares 13g of the 85% dark chocolate with 25g of black raisins, a ~500cal meal. Mmm, I'm going to make that, NCD Bunless Burger & Chocolate Raisins!

I mean. Do you really want a white hamburger bun? No you don't. The inner you doesn't at least. Many people eat carbs mindlessly, never understanding what a carb is for. It's for energy. And if you've got body fat, then you've got energy sitting there waiting to be used. And you can't eat the white bun AND have the raisins. You have to pick-and-choose your carbs. And your first choice should be from plants. Since most vegetables are free, except, peas (and beans), corn, potatoes, sweet potatoes, yams, and pumpkin, your other choices for carbs with colors, is Fruit.

On the NCD we make fruit a part of our meal, so that we eat less bread, rice, and pasta.

NCD Three "Starch" Categories™
1. sprouted bread, true whole grains, and occasional enriched
2. potatoes, peas, corn, sweet potatoes, yams, pumpkin, and beans
3. fruit, fresh, dried, juice, and the NCD Healthy Sugars™

It's that last one that makes this diet different from most others. But then the other diets will tell you you can't have fruit. Or, if they allow fruit, it's five small strawberries, oooh, 30 calories. By "others" I am referring to the majority of the diets out there which are based on cutting carbs, the slow-carb, low-carb, no-carb diets. It works. That's why it's popular. But, like I said before, at a certain point you run the risk of going back to your old way of eating because sooner or later you're going to want a glass of orange juice or a banana or a bowl of grapes. Then your DI says, "Ah, thank God, I'm so low in here I could barely keep things running, gimme some more." And you do, and do and do and do, until you've undone everything.

The other aspect of the NCD that makes it different from the others is the FREEDOM to eat what you want and the FLEXIBILITY to adapt to fat loss, muscle gain, or weight maintenance, and to your lifestyle, six meals a day or three double meals a day. And the chocolate! I forgot the chocolate! You get to be Bad as well as be Good. It's really The Fantasy Diet!™ The All Your Dreams Come True Diet!

But first we have to get past the math part. You'll get it. You've seen all the calculations, we're just repeating it over-and-over with different food items, portion sizes, and recipes.

CHAPTER 27

Taco Seasoning

There are two seasonings that you will make from scratch at home, this one and the Italian Seasoning. Both are so easy to make and you will not encounter any undesirables found in store-bought packaged seasonings.

This taco seasoning will also be used in the NCD Hard Shell Tacos™ recipe, and if you want to do one low-carb meal a day to speed up fat loss, one way is to substitute a 40 30 30 meal with 500 calories of peanuts. Plain peanuts are 4% carbs with the fiber subtracted, and 18% protein to sustain you. This is a great way to cut your carbs. And who doesn't like peanuts! When you get bored of having them plain, we switch to hot-and-spicy NCD Chili Peanuts™. BUT, that's a big but for a reason, BUT, don't do more than one peanut-meal substitution per day. Otherwise, you'll be on a low-carb slow-carb no-carb diet, and we already know where that usually ends up.

So, I never got to this in the ABC NCD. We did discuss the NCD One Fruit Meal™ option for the person who wants to feed their muscles and gain size, 40 30 30 x5, and one 500cal fruit 'meal', so now we have the NCD One Nocarb Meal™ for the person whose goal is to cut fat. Assuming 2500 calories, you'll have 4 meals of 40 30 30 and one proFat 'meal'. Small "p" because 18% is a little low. We'll get to all that. But for now, we're going to make Taco Seasoning. Olé!

OMG! Just for the record, I don't provide references or citations because this should make sense to you. The principles and statements etc., should ring true. If your Divine Intelligence is working, it should recognize common-sense truth. That said, there are times when I fact-check. Some material I know off the top of my head, back-side-front, as I have taken the subject matter and created my own reference binders. Other times, I have to check one of the books I've read, which is so easy to do when they're all filed by the year I read them, and the chapters of the books are all tabbed with those peel-and-stick index tabs you can buy at Office Max (I've spent a small fortune on those tabs, but if you're OCD like I am then you must have them). Other times, I go to the internet to look up the current spelling of a word (my, how spelling has changed since I did my undergraduate English and Linguistics classes back in the 80s), or to find out what Splenda really is, etc.

Anyway, olé originates from the Arabic word wallah, which means "by God". OMG! Who knew.

So what I should have said was…But for now, we're going to make some Taco Seasoning. Ándale!

There is also not a lot of agreement when it comes to certain word spellings and usages. You have undoubtedly noticed my style of writing and I explained why I do things the way I do in the "Edits & Format" section at the beginning. Capitalizing every Pyrex, Walmart, SKS, and AKA, just gets to be too much. Then when I need to get your attention, like with my big BUT, it would get missed. Can not and cannot are two usages that you may not be aware of, I wasn't. Can not means, the possibility exists, but you "must not". Whereas, cannot means, there is no possibility, it's not possible. My writing style is for the purpose of communicating the information from me to you, I'm not writing a scientific paper for peer review or filling out an application for a grant. All that to say this. I am checking my facts, and you are welcome to check them as well.

So, Ándale! Let's go! Óle! Oh my God!

137

You will need nine spices. I've replaced many of my regular supermarket-brand spices with organic spices from the healthfood store, no pesticides. They cost practically the same amount. So just toss your old ones and switch over.

Spices are antioxidants, remember the champion? Curcumin. The yellow color found in Turmeric, used in Curry. You can purchase curcumin as a supplement, but not as a spice, as it's a spice extract. I call it a spice so that the government doesn't decide to re-categorize it as a drug, since curcumin is also anti-inflammatory. Curcumin has so many positive healing properties that I am sure drug companies are itching to own it. If you haven't set up your shakers of Turmeric and Curry, and ground Cloves, do so now. Spices are Time Test – Pass. You can purchase curcumin capsules at bioinnovations.net, but don't try to open the capsule and sprinkle it onto your food as its yellow color will stain everything yellow.

There is power in those plant colors.

So our nine taco seasonings in descending order by amount, are:

1. 4T 26g Red Pepper Powder, aka, red chili pepper, cayenne
2. 2T 12g Ground Cumin, (not curcumin), cumin's brown
3. 4t 20g Sea Salt
4. 4t 11g Ground Black Pepper, finely ground is best
5. 2t 5g Paprika – I'm using cedar-wood smoked paprika
6. 1t 4g Garlic Powder
7. 1t 2g Onion Powder – not onion salt or onion flakes
8. 1t 2g Red Pepper Flakes – red chili pepper, for pizzas
9. 1t 0g Oregano

If you are new to cooking and you've never used spices like these before, I was the same at one time. I never used spices because I didn't know when and where to use them. Just go buy these, look at them, open them up, smell them, taste them a little bit, and you will quickly come to know the differences and what each of them does. Some of them are obvious when you smell them. Oregano says SPAGHETTI SAUCE! Cumin says warm soups and Mexican meals. Red pepper powder for heat. Actually, one of my favorite spices is just black pepper. Maybe that's why it's on the table at every restaurant. NCD Chicken Caesar Salad™ with freshly ground black pepper, mmm, it doesn't get any better than that.

As you can see I've given you the amount in grams so all you have to do is place a bowl on the scale, turn it on, add 26 grams of red pepper powder, press tare to zero it, add 12g of cumin, zero it, add 20g of salt, press tare, 11g of black pepper, and keep going until you've done all 8. The 1t of oregano didn't weigh anything so you can use a measuring spoon or eyeball it. Whisk it to mix it, and transfer it to an 8oz sks jar with screw cap. Label it and refrigerate. I refrigerate all my spices. They're foods with nutrients.

The no-bowl method. This is my preferred way. Place an 8oz sks jar on the scale, zero it, add 26g of red pepper powder, zero it, add 12g cumin, zero it, etc., all the way to the end, then cap and shake. No bowl or whisk to wash.

If you don't own, or want to use, a scale, well, measure away.

For the 12-meal taco salad, we will use 20g for medium kick, 15g for med-mild, and 10g for mild. DO NOT go higher than 20g.

NCD Spicy Rule™
Spice to Medium at the most. Never to Hot.

You see, hot spice, overly-hot spice, inflames your colon walls. Inflammation is followed by bleeding. GI Bleed. Working in a hospital for 20 years, there was usually one GI-bleed patient a week. And how do you stop a 15-foot long colon from bleeding? Well, you give them blood products, and when that no longer works, you take them to surgery, and well, the outcome is usually not good. If you live in a rural area, your local hospital may not stock a lot of blood products, so you bleed-out before they can get you to the big hospital. Hot in your mouth means burning and bleeding on the way down to the other end. In fact, Walmart has taken Hot Picante Sauce off their shelves. You don't need hot.

The second thing that hot spice does to the colon is, it wipes away all your good bacteria. So now your digestion is off. And by off, I mean, your food doesn't digest and you have those embarrassing moments. Certain cultures of people need to go easy on the spice for this very reason. If you have flatulence after a meal with spice, it was too hot.

In fact, certain people believe that the hot-spicy food is killing "germs" in their colon. It is. But the answer is not to kill germs with hot spice, the answer is to not consume germs! See, JPM Nontoxic Hand Sanitizer & Hand Towelettes in *Nontoxic Teeth Whitening and Dental Hygiene System*.

It's better to make this dish with the 10 grams of taco seasoning, mild, then if you want a bit more spice you can add a bit more at the table.

Spices are concentrated. You don't need a lot.

To help you memorize this seasoning recipe, here's a list of "five".

1. Cumin, the taco spice
2. Red Chili Pepper – Powder & Flakes.
3. Salt & Pepper
4. Garlic & Onion – powders for both
5. Oregano & Paprika – O&P

Okay! Let's make that Taco Salad!

Chapter Endnote
You are going to see some abbreviated word forms and new words coming up. If you see an "x" in front of a word, read it as "extra". Note, "lowercarb" and "lowcarb". Lowercarb refers to a tweak from 40 to 30%, whereas lowcarb implies a shift to atkins, 20-10% carbs. The word "dipwashing" sounds, yes, retarded, BUT, it accurately describes and gives you a clear visual picture of the washing movement. Let's Go!

CHAPTER 28

The Anabolic Effect

Step 1 – the chips
If you bought the 4 bags of chips for 24 taco salads, do all 4 now.
Grab 6 xsmall pyrex bowls and one bag of chips. Crush the chips
in the bag with your hands, open the bag and aliquot the chips into
the 6 bowls, 1.2oz per bowl. You can place a bowl on the scale,
add 1.2oz of chips, and now you have a visual reference, and then
eyeball the remainder. They may give you a bit more than 7oz per
bag, so you may end up with 1.3oz in some of them. Repeat this
again and again and again for bags 2, 3, and 4. Chips are done.

Step 2 – the cheese
Grab a large pyrex bowl and the 12oz cheddar. Place a cheese
grater in the bowl and shred your cheddar cheese. Cover and
refrigerate. If you bought two 12oz cheddar for 24 meals, do the
second cheddar now, in a separate large pyrex bowl, for next week.
If you are going to be taking this salad to work, transfer 1.0oz of
the shredded cheese to an xsmall pyrex bowl. Cheese is done.

Step 3 – the romaine
Fill an xlarge bowl with hot water, or use a rinsed and towel-wiped
sink. Grab one romaine head and break off 2-3 leaves. "Dip
Wash" the leaves six times, submerge them into the hot water, pull
them out, submerge and out, four more times. Flick the leaves
after they come out of the sixth dipwash and place them in a
colander. Continue doing this dipwashing of your lettuce leaves

until your first head of romaine is done. Now drain the water and repeat the process for the second head of romaine. Then drain the water and do the 3rd head, then drain and do the 4th head.

So, we dipwash the leaves 6x in hot water, 2-3 leaves at a time, and start with a fresh sink of hot water for each head of romaine.

This might seem like a lot, but you've got to get those pesticides off, and hot water is the best way to do it. The movement itself, submerge-and-up, submerge-and-up, is also very effective for removing pesticides. So, the hot water combined with the up-and-down washing movement will do the trick. The time in the hot water will be about six seconds, and-one and-two and-three and-four and-five and-six, flick, place aside, start again. After a while you'll just realize that it's just what you have to do if you are going to eat nonorganic lettuce. Also, any *E. coli* and *Salmonella* that periodically contaminates spinach and lettuce will be removed too.

You get to skip your NCD Leafy Green Protocol™ this week, that's the good news!

Lastly, examine your leaves and use a scissors to cut off any black edges or brown spots. Break and tear the leaves up with your hands and add 6oz to each of 12 large pyrex rectangles (or bowls).

Step 4 – the beans
The day before, add 4t 21g of salt to a half-gallon glass bottle, like the one-gallon bottles for the ABC Water, but a half gallon. Then, add 1900g of pH 7.5 water. Remember, we need the water to be alkaline or our beans will not soften, but too much baking soda and they will be too soft. If you follow this procedure, your beans will come out perfect. Cap and mix your pH-7.5 21g-salt water. Refrigerate overnight. This allows it to completely dissolve. Just because it looks dissolved that doesn't mean it is. Good cooking means good mixing.

Next day. Pour the salt water into a 6qt crockpot. Add 100g of your pH-7.5 water to the empty half-gallon bottle, swirl, and add it to the crockpot = 2000g of water total. If you do this right, you won't have to drain any excess water from the beans at the end, pouring some of your bean nutrients down the drain.

Rinse the kidney beans in a bowl and then dump them into a colander, do this three times. There is never any dirt, so you could do this one time if you want. Take your colander of kidney beans and add them to the crockpot. Spread them out. You want the kidney beans on the bottom and the black beans on top because the kidney beans require more heat to cook them than the black beans. Rinse the black beans 1-3x and add them to the crockpot in a layer on top of the kidney beans. Cover and cook on low for six hours.

Tip. Buy a timer-outlet from Walmart for $10. Set the time, and then program the timer to start now, and end in six hours. Plug the crockpot into the timer, and plug the timer into the wall outlet. Now you are free to do as you please. The crockpot will shut off automatically in six hours. It can sit overnight, that's fine as well.

In the morning, or when it's done and cooled off some, add half to an XXlarge flat-bottom bowl, and the other half to a large pyrex bowl for next week. If you are making 12 meals, then use one bag of beans, either the kidney or the black, and add the entire amount to the XXlarge bowl. Use half the water (1000g) for one bag of beans, and you will have to adjust your cooking time down a bit.

Step 5 – the tomatoes
If you are doing 24 salads, you will repeat this step next week. We don't want the tomatoes sitting in the refrigerator for a week. Open the big can of tomatoes, add half the can to the XXlarge bowl, add half of your remaining half to a wave blender. Add 20g of taco seasoning for medium, or 10g for mild. Blend. Add the remaining tomatoes to the blender and blend again. Pour this into the XXlarge bowl. This way your seasoning is thoroughly mixed.

A wave blended is a must-have. The pitcher has a groove in it so the contents shoot up the side and then down onto the blade. Ingenious. I have the Hamilton Beach Wave Maker Blender.

Unfortunately, you may not be able to find them because this $15 blender made all the other expensive old-style blenders worthless, including those super-expensive $250 models. So, instead of the old style disappearing, somebody must have said, "Get rid of that wave blender, or it will put our company out of business." So this ingenious invention has slowly disappeared from the shelves.

Step 6 – the beef

Add 2.5 packs 2.5lbs of the ground beef to a large skillet. Place the remaining 8oz in a flip-top sandwich bag and then into a vacuum-seal bag and vacuum seal it for next week. If you are making 12 meals, then cook the three pounds and pull off 1/6th of it at the end. Break the ground beef apart with a turner spatula and mix-and-flip the beef as it cooks. Don't walk away. Stay there, breaking it apart and mixing and flipping it until it's MW, slight pink remaining. Unplug the skillet and continue to mix-and-flip off heat until the pink just disappears, and then add it to the XXlarge bowl. Perfect.

Step 7 – aliquoting

Stir the contents of your XXlarge bowl and aliquot it into twelve 16oz sks jars, 16oz 454g each, full to the top. To get this step right, weigh your XXlarge bowl empty. Write it down. Then weigh your bowl of chili. Subtract the weight of the bowl and divide by 12. That is the weight of each serving of chili.

A twist. At one time a 10-pound capacity kitchen scale was the highest you could buy. Now, Walmart has 20 pounds and even one with a 35-pound capacity. Unfortunately, they are battery operated. Having a 20 or 35 pound capacity scale is useful because this batch of chili weighs 12 lbs, and the bowl weighs 1.7 lbs, 13.7 lbs total. When this happens, I weigh the batch in two parts to determine the total weight of the batch. Then add them together and divide by 12. Presently, this chili done this way weighs 5445g total, divided by 12 = 454g per serving. If you bought the SKS jars, it's a 16oz jar full to the top, and the screw cap allows it to last ~10 days.

Are you ready for some taco salad! I should say so! This recipe is a bit of work that's true, but let's quickly look at the Pros and Cons.

Cons. It's a bit time-consuming and there's some work involved and there are some dishes to wash, the skillet, the crockpot, and let's not forget about that dipwashing.

Pros. When you have finished the week and eaten your 12 taco salads, you will have consumed, 6.4 pounds of tomatoes, RED, a pound of kidney or black beans, 4 heads of DARK LEAFY GREENS, 3/4^{ths} pound of raw cheese probiotics, 2.5 pounds of ground beef, 2 bags of baked organic blue corn chips, and a bunch of different spices. On top of that, this meal is very satisfying, very nutritious, well worth the work, and ANABOLIC.

Yes. Recall how in the ABC NCD we talked about anabolism kicking-in after a meal, page 106. Your muscles just start to expand, much like the Incredible Hulk character. This salad does that for me. It's really more like the NCD Anabolic Taco Salad. And it's a lot cheaper and safer than steroids, not to mention legal.

You'll get faster each time you make it. Oh, and one more Pro. All that nutrition and quality for $2.44. You'll never eat a Taco Salad this good in any restaurant. They don't have the right numbers.

E=524   (130+110+50+63+63+108)
F=133   (18+80+2+33)
Na=1172   (189+170+756+57) (plus the seasoning Na)
CHO=230   (104+32+47+47)
f=48   (9+8+12+19)
s=28   (24+2+2)
Prot=157   (14+28+8+17+16+74)
T=520   T-f=472
44 26 30   39 28 33
Our protein is stable at 30% or 33. Our carbs and fats are just fine. Post-meal feel is fantastic. It's perfect as is.

To serve it, cover the jar of chili with a paper towel and microwave it 1min + 30sec + 30sec, or if the weather is hot, 1m + 30s. Sprinkle the crushed chips on top of the romaine, pour the hot chili on top, sprinkle with 1.0oz cheddar. Mmm, Enjoy!

CHAPTER 29

NCD Peanuts™

Let's do the low carb no carb proFat. The NCD macros for a ProFat, capital P, are with the protein still at 30%, so 150 calories of protein. Then, there's about 50 calories of carbs, and the fat is double, 150 calories x2 = 300 calories.

Carbs = 50 cal
Fat = 300 cal
Prot = 150 cal
T = 500

50/500x100=10% 300/500x100=60% 150/500x100=30%

NCD ProFat Meal™
10 60 30
10% carbs 60% fat 30% protein

You are permitted to do ONE low-carb meal substitution per day, or every-other-day, or every day every-other-week. Absolute maximum of two substitutions per day, short term only.

I have done the two ProFat meals and three 40 30 30 meals a day, but only for 1-3 days, BUT, you have to have good energy and mood to do it. If you are tired and a bit irritable, your carb cutting won't work. You'll just become a step more tired and a bit more irritable. It's easy to tell when someone's on a low-carb diet.

Again, if you are trying to create an anabolic effect and make your muscles grow and expand, low carb is not going to do it. Unless you're a 20-year-old male in great physical shape with skyrocketing T and GH, testosterone and growth hormone. If this is you, you can eat just about any way you want and work out and get results. But, eventually, you'll be 30, and 40, and 50.

Don't get greedy with wanting the fat to come off. Just get the ball rolling, and then stick to it and get busy with life. NCD Kitchen Closed at Five™ is still one of the best ways to wake up each morning thinner and leaner. Nothing 3-4-5 hours before bed. Also, "get busy with life" means, Move, Work, Walk, Hustle, not sit.

So, our peanuts have 91 calories 18% protein and so they are a proFat, small "p", a bit lower than our 150cal 30% target. None-the-less, they are great for cutting carbs, and so easy to "make".

1. Old-Fashioned Blister Peanuts, unsalted
TJs brand 13oz 368g $4.69 buy 3 bags. Extra large water blanched Virginia peanuts, peanut oil. The nutrition facts say,
1/4cup 30g servings about 12
E=180
F=140
CHO=5g
Prot=8g
Try to find one that matches this, or higher protein, but not lower. We are going to make 13 proFat meals.

Step 1
Add the 3 bags to a big bowl. Grab 13, 6oz sks jars and place one on the scale. Fill it with 3.0oz of peanuts (85g), repeat 12x more. When you get near the end, dump the remaining peanuts into a colander that has big holes and shake it to remove the little round hard pieces. Then continue filling your last couple of jars, and there you have it, 13 servings of 3.0oz peanuts. Cap & Refrigerate.

If you take the time to remove those little ball-like pieces of peanuts using the colander, you will enjoy your peanuts more and they will look nicer in the jar. Remember, this is your meal for the next 2-3-4 hours so make it special.

For the NCD Chili Peanuts™, before capping, add one level 1/8th measuring teaspoon to each jar. Or, do 6 spicy and leave 7 plain. If you add the spice to the 3 bags of peanuts in the bowl, then it gets a bit messy. So just scoop-and-swipe scoop-and-swipe your 1/8th measuring spoon and you'll be done in less-than a minute. I usually make the first batch of 13 plain, and then when I make it again, I do 13 spicy. 1/8t will make it mild. You don't want to go more than mild as you will be having this every day for the next 13 days, so spicier will burn out your normal colon flora by day 5. So keep it mild and 13 servings will not harm your good gut bacteria.

Aside. A nurse once challenged me on my use of the word "flora" on a Gram-Stain report.   Check any medical-microbiology textbook, I have two thick ones, microbiologist call bacteria populations "flora". She insisted it was strictly used for flowers.

Our final numbers are, 3oz 85g peanuts,
E=510
F=396
SF=76
Na=0
CHO=57   nCHO=23
f=34
s=91
Prot=91
T=544   T-f=510
10.5 72.8 16.7 rounded to 10 73 17 with nCHO it's 4 78 18.
So, 10.5% carbs, and with the fiber subtracted, 4% carbs.
The satfat is 76/544x100=14%. Peanuts are mostly omega-9, OAP.

The protein of 91 calories 18% is good, it will sustain you. The fat will fill you up, and they taste great. This is your Go-To low-carb substitute. You can do it for 13 days, then do the NCD Tuna Guacamole™, then 13 days of peanuts again, then the NCD Ham & Havarti™, then 13 days of peanuts. Then back to all 40 30 30 meals for a while. You will have cut carbs for 8 weeks, and you won't have even noticed it, much. I wouldn't keep doing this, as your desire for other foods will grow, so do the 8 weeks and then wait 4 months and then do the 8 weeks again. That would be twice a year. Or, you could do 4 weeks 4 times a year, every third month.

NCD Lowercarb Cycle™
Jan Feb – 8 weeks 40 30 30 x4 plus one p/ProFat meal
Mar April May June – 40 30 30 x5
July Aug – 8 weeks 40 30 30 x4 plus one p/ProFat meal
Sept Oct Nov Dec – 40 30 30 x5

NCD Fat Cutting Tools™
1. NCD Lowercarb Cycle – as above
2. NCD Kitchen Closed at Five, 3-4-5 hours before bed
3. Sporadically omit a portion of the carbs with any 40 30 30 meal
4. NCD Recalibration Exercise, cross-country-ski walking
5. NCD Free Vegetables – see ABC NCD, NCD Grapefruit™

Do you see how uncrazy this is? If you use these 5 tools, the fat will come off, and then melt off, and then you're there.

The NCD – a Unique Approach to Weight Management™
Bridging You From Advice to Results – JPM

BUT, first you have to get control of the numbers you're eating by eating pre-counted meals and keeping track of them.

If you don't have a daily planner, one with half a page for each day so you can make notes, then make one or buy one. I like to have one sheet per day, double-sided. I make my own. I fold it in half, so it's the size of a book, it fits right inside the cover of whatever book I happen to be reading, and I take it with me everywhere I go. On the inside, it has a 24-hour day, and that's where I record my activities, meals, exercise, my vegetable snacks, cardio, everything. On the outside is my "To Do" list and reminders. So I use this to track. And I suggest you do the same, use whatever version you like, but track.

NCD T=>C=>R Strategy™
What doesn't get tracked doesn't get controlled doesn't get results.

Or, you can be out of control with your weight and eating, or up and down, it's up to you. The NCD is about having freedom and choice. We have lots of freedom to eat whatever we like and choose whatever we want, but with COMPLETE CONTROL over the whole thing.

Yes, I'm a control freak. With OCD. And a sense of humor!

Seriously though, think of your body as a business. You have to manage it, organize it, track it, and work it, if you want it to be in tip-top shape into your 50s 60s 70s and 80s. Many people's bodies fizzle out and "go-out-of-business" as they approach their 60s and 70s, or younger. It's true. Science has determined that, when compared to other animals and species, a human should live to be 120. This would mean that many of us are living to just a little past the halfway mark. Your next question should be, Why?

CHAPTER 30

NCD Guac & Tuna™

Again, understand that I abbreviate things for simplicity. You get it. I don't need to spell out Chocolate or Carbohydrate or Guacamole every time. And I use unique words and spellings.

So, the title tells you what you'll be eating. This recipe is a true ProFat, with 133 calories of protein providing 27 or 32% protein per meal.

The recipe makes 2, so you can double it and make 4, or triple it and make 6. Let's assume it's July and the last time you made this recipe was in January, 6 months ago, see our lowercarb cycle in the previous chapter. Since it's been 6 months, let's quadruple the recipe and make 8. If we do 13 days of peanuts and 8 days of this, we will have 21 days, 3 weeks.

I sometimes stock those peanuts in my refrigerator so that if I run out of 40 30 30 meals because I'm busy, I have the peanuts instead of fastfood. Heads-up, I have a few fastfood restaurant options for emergencies, so stay tuned for that. And don't forget about our 1qt of 2% milk NCD Emergency Meal™ (main book, page 272).

If you want to, you can do 15 days of peanuts and 6 days of this recipe = 21 days, or, 5 peanuts and 2 of this, times 3wks = 21 days.

I am doing 8 meals so I need 8 cans of tuna and 4lbs of guacamole.

1. Tongol Chunk Light Tuna, in water, no salt added
TJs brand, 6.5oz 184g, drained weight 4.7oz 133g, $1.69 x8 cans.
Ingredients, tuna, water. It's wild caught and dolphin safe, from
Thailand. It also says that in Europe it is called white tuna, like
Albacore, because it meets their spectrographic tests. And yes,
when you open it, it's not brown like chunk light tuna but more of
a pale tan color.

2oz 56g servings about 2.5 drained
E=60
F=5
Prot=14g
Try to find one like this, most tuna in water are. We will use the
entire can, drained, 133g/56g=2.38, so we multiply our NF label by
2.38, E=143 F=12 Na=119 CHO=0 Prot=133 T=145, 0 8 92.
This tuna is nearly 100% protein, 92%, and 8% fat, fish fat, good
hormones.

Note, a 5oz can of tuna has 118 calories of protein, that's fine, or a
6oz can is good.

2. Guacamole
TJs brand, 16oz 1lb 454g (two 8oz pouches) $3.99, buy 4. This is
the guacamole in the cardboard box with two plastic containers or
pouches. Many stores have dropped the size to 14oz with two 7oz
pouches. TJs is the only place that hasn't dropped the size. Try to
find the 16oz box, and if they don't have it, ask the store manager
why the sizes are getting smaller and call the 800 number on the
back, let them know the customer is watching and paying attention.

Ingredients, hass avocados, tomato, onion, jalapeño pepper, serrano
pepper, salt, cilantro, garlic. I've made guacamole from scratch
before and it's so much better, but you have to find ripe avocados,
and it is a bit of work. But if you have time, make your own. The
other option is, to buy guacamole sides at Chipotle restaurant for
$1.25 per 4oz, x4=16oz for $5, plus tax. It's this guacamole green
plant fat that your body really wants, so load up on it and you will
find, "You don't really want guacamole and chips."

Product Information. If there is information on the product, the NCD says you have to read it. Start to do so and you'll be amazed at how much you'll learn. This guacamole says, "Did you know that throughout history avocado has been known as a powerful aphrodisiac? We can attest that, at the very least, our moods have improved." So there you go. You can toss both your Viagra and Prozac in the trash.

We saw in the ABC NCD that walnuts are shaped round like your head, and the nut is convoluted like the surface of your brain. If you slice a carrot from the end and look at one of the slices, it's a circle shape with radial rings, like your eye. A sweet potato on the counter is how your pancreas sits inside your body. Place a stock of celery on the counter with the bottom pointing at you and the top pointing ahead of you, then look down at your feet. Celery stocks and rhubarb stocks look like the bones in your body. Place an olive with part of the branch attached, and another one next to it east and west, and you have the ovaries. A bundle of grapes look like the round alveolar sacs of the lungs. We all know that kidney beans are shaped like the kidneys. A tomato cut in half has chambers much like the heart. Well, the avocado hangs like the male testicles, and flip it upside down and it sits like the female uterus.

The NCD encourages you to choose God's foods over man-made foods – because they resemble the human anatomy.

You will use one 8oz pouch of guacamole. If you can only find the 14oz box then the 7oz pouch is fine. 2T 30g E=45 F=35, so 8oz 227g is E=341 F=265 SF=68 Na=757 CHO=91 f=91 s=0 Prot=0 T=356, 26 74 0. T-f=265, 0 100 0. SF=19% (it's an omega-9).

So, with the fiber subtracted, the carbs are zero, and this becomes a 100%-fat food. 91 calories of fiber is 23 grams, that's 77% of your daily-recommended fiber per meal!

Tip. If you ever have…yeah, that, constipation. Oils and fats work so much better than Metamucil and all those other over-the-counter things. We'll come back to this during the parasite cleanse. But, suffice-it-to-say, this meal has a nice clearing effect on the colon. Surely you've noticed how energetic a dog or a cat is, or a coworker is, after they've come back from the restroom. A full colon robs you of energy. A full colon is more likely to prevent you from exercising and working out, or from simply doing household chores.

Step 1

Remove the 8 pouches of guacamole from the boxes, toss the boxes in the recycler and place the pouches on the shelf in your refrigerator. Place the 8 cans of tuna next to it. This way, your brain doesn't have to think about what to eat. The meal is right there saying, "I'm right here, make me!" This will prevent you from saying, "Uh, I'll just open a bag of chips or go to McDonalds."

The key is to have everything you need for your meal all in one spot.™

If it's not grab-and-go in one place, you will opt for something else that's comforting and familiar. So buy that freezerless refrigerator with the 5 shelves and place breakfast meals on the top, boom, everything you need in one spot to put it together, 2-5 minutes and you're ready to eat, lunches on shelf 2, dinners on shelf 3, ABC Water on shelf 4, and miscellaneous items on the bottom, shelf 5.

So this is why the cans of tuna are in the refrigerator.

You need to make your "Meal Making Mindless" otherwise you'll opt for something easier. If it's too spread out in different areas of your kitchen, you'll be less likely to "Get-A-Visual" of the meal and put it together.

Time to eat!

Open one can of tuna, drain it and squeeze it. If you don't like the taste of fish, squeeze out the liquid until it is very dry and you won't be able to taste it. Using a fork, add the tuna to a big cereal bowl and fluff it up. Add one 8oz pouch or 7oz tray of guacamole and mix it with the tuna.   Sit down, Pray, to change your physiology from "doing" to "eating", and eat it with a fork. It's quite good. It just seems plain because it's missing the carbs.

Our final numbers are,
E=484
F=277
Na=876
CHO=91   nCHO=0
f=91
s=0
Prot=133
T=501 18 55 27   T-f=410 0 68 32
So our protein is 27 or 32%, and "no" carbs, and the rest is fat, 68%. This is a NCD ProFat. Price per serving, $3.69.

Our net calories are 410, 90 less-than 500. If your energy drops an hour-and-a-half later, you could have 3 squares 10g of our 85% Green & Black's dark chocolate = 63 calories.

3sq 10g 85% dark chocolate
E=63 F=45 Na=3 CHO=15 f=4 s=8 Prot=4 T=64

So our variation is the NCD GuacTuna & Choc™.
E=574
F=322
Na=879
CHO=106   nCHO=11
f=95
s=8
Prot=137
T=565 19 57 24   T-f=470 2 69 29
So with the fiber subtracted, which we need to do because the guacamole is 26% fiber, our calories are 470, our macros are 2% carbs, 8 calories of sugar, so basically nothing, 69% fat, and 29% protein. Excellent. The theobromine in the cocoa will give you energy and keep you in a good mood!

CHAPTER 31

NCD Ham & Havarti™

So we've done 3 weeks of the NCD Lowercarb Cycle, 13 days of peanuts and 8 days of tuna-guacamole & chocolate. Let's do the peanuts again, your "go-to" low-carb meal, but let's make them with the 1/8t of taco seasoning with each serving. The peanuts have a slight bit of oil, as the ingredients said peanuts and peanut oil, so all you do is add a level 1/8t taco seasoning, cap-and-shake, and they will be evenly coated. Spicy Peanuts!

So for this recipe we will do 10 days, that will bring us to 13+8+13+10=44 days, then finish the cycle with 13 days of plain peanuts, 44+13=57 days, or 8 weeks plus a day, 13-peanuts + 8-guactuna + 13-peanuts + 10-hamhavarti + 13-peanuts = 8 weeks.

1. Harvarti Sliced Cheese
TJs brand 10oz 238g $3.99 buy 3. Pasteurized milk, cheese cultures, salt, microbial rennet, cows not treated with rBST. Recombinant Bovine Somatotropin hormone. Hm, doesn't sound like anything God made. So, the NCD says avoid it. Isn't it odd that in the 1990s when all the milk at your average supermarket had rBST, that at the same time mothers where finding it equally odd that their daughters were developing breasts at the age of nine and ten? It was probably just a coincidence.

One slice 1oz 28g E=110 F=80 SF=6gx9=54cal Na=210 CHO=0 Prot=6gx4=24cal T=104, 0 77 23, and SF is 54/104x100=52%.

So again, cheese is a 77% fat food and 52% saturated fat. What percent of the FAT is Saturated Fat? Tick tick tick tick, 54/80x100, saturated-fat cals over fat cals x100=67.5% or 68%. So this is not an omega 3, 6 or 9 fat. It's a saturated fat, 68% of the fat is saturated fat. We eat both, plant fat and animal fat, on the NCD.

We need a balance of all fats. The ones people are missing though are Omega-3 Flax Seeds and Fish Fat DHA and EPA.

We will have 3oz 3 slices per meal. That sounds like a lot, but that's what low carb is, your body runs on fat for fuel instead of carbs. It works fine, it just gets boring without the carbs.

Suppose you were going to eat 2000 calories a day, 4 meals of 500 calories spaced 4-hours apart.
06:00 Up
07:00 Breakfast   40 30 30 500cal
11:00 Lunch   40 30 30 500cal
15:00 ProFat Meal   500cal
19:00 Dinner   40 30 30 500cal
22:00 lights out

You could easily lose fat. Firstly, you had 200 calories of carbs at 11:00, and then no carbs for 8 hours until 19:00. Then, you had 200 calories of carbs at 19:00, and no carbs until 07:00 the following day, that's 12 hours. So, within your 24-hour day, you have two carb fasts, one of 8 hours, and one of 12 hours. Plus, your total carb intake for the 24 hours is 600 calories, or 150g. 600 divided by 2000 x100 = 30%. You've dropped your carbs from 40% to 30%. DON'T add exercise or you'll become carb depleted after a week. Just stay busy and get used to the lower carbs.

Then, after your NCD Lowercarb Cycle is over in 8 weeks, you go back to 40 30 30 x4 meals a day and throw in 30-45 minutes of the walking. You will still be losing fat.

Later on, start taking boot camp high-intensity cardio classes, or better yet, the cardio-weights classes, aka, interval training, where you do cardio, then you lift weights, then back to cardio, then weights. Add 250 calories to your diet at the beginning. Then, as you get in shape and start to sweat and you finish the class with the back of your shirt wet, then add another 250 calories and eat 2500 per day. This is where you will see your body TRANSFORM.

It takes MUSCLE to burn calories. In fact, your calories are being burned by your MUSCLES. So use them. And the harder you use them the more you will burn calories, think, Anaerobic Exercise.

NCD Fat Loss Alternative™
Stay on maintenance calories, just add Weights & Cardio.

Suppose you just can't cut back on your eating. Fine. Stay on maintenance calories. But add to your week as many weights-and-cardio sessions as you can, without overdoing it to the point that you want to eat more. Intense exercise makes a person hungry afterwards, so plan your exercise so that it ends 30-45 minutes before your next meal, i.e., the class ends at 18:30, you shower and drive home and make something to eat at 19:00-19:15, 19:30 at the latest.

When your goal is to lose fat, then you have to plan your meals and time them, and pay close attention. Why? Because you are in a calorie deficit. Your body needs 3000 but you're only giving it 2500. Or, you need 2500 and you're only giving it 2000.

The preferred fat loss method is to keep your calories the same, but add Weights & Cardio to your lifestyle.

But you have to get your calories under control. That's the first step. The average everyday person has no accurate idea of how many calories they eat. But this won't be you!

The 3 slices 3oz of cheese is E=330 F=240 Na=610 Prot=72 T=312.

You can use swiss or cheddar or pepper jack, whichever you prefer.

We will use the other cheeses elsewhere, so here's where I like to have Havarti.   If you never had Havarti cheese before, it's delicious. It's originally from Denmark so many people have never tasted it. Swiss goes good with this as well, so you can buy 2 swiss and 1 havarti, or 1 swiss, 1 havarti, and 1 cheddar, colby, or pepper jack. All 1oz servings of cheese, (regular cheese not reduced fat), are usually E=110 F=80. If you buy a 12oz 12 slice pack, then buy two packs and make 8 meals, 12x2=24 slices ÷ 3 = 8 meals.

2. Healthy Ham
TJs market, Celebrity brand, 8oz 227g $2.49, buy 1 package for every 2 meals, so for 10 meals buy 5 packs. We will use half the pack, 4oz per meal. No ingredients listed, just the "cured with" list of salts, same as the canadian-bacon for the Hawaiian Pizza. It's the same company and it has the AHA heart emblem with the 50% less sodium, and it says 99% fat free.

1 slice 28g servings per container 8
E=20
F=0
CHO=0
Prot=5g
Try to find one like this. Look for 99% fat free on the front label. Half the package is 4oz 4 slices E=80 F=0 Na=720 CHO=0 Prot=80 T=80, 0 0 100. It's no carbs no fat 100% protein. Nice. There's probably a little fat in it, but it is lean. If you can only find 97% fat-free or 96% fat-free ham, then buy half of your cheese as reduced fat and half as regular, then use 1.5 slices of reduced-fat cheese and 1.5 slices of regular-fat cheese with each meal.

We are going to make ROLL-UPS! Ham and Havarti Roll-ups!

Take 4 slices of ham and 3 slices of cheese. Place 1 slice of cheese on top of 1 slice of ham and roll it from end to end. Repeat with the second slice of cheese. For the third slice of cheese you will roll it up with 2 slices of ham. Now you have 3 ham-and-cheese roll-ups, two with 1 slice of ham and one with 2 slices of ham. Two will be more cheesy than ham, and one will be more hammy than cheese. Variety. Fun. If you do one with a slice of swiss, one with a slice of cheddar, and one with a slice of havarti, then you have even more variety. More fun!

Bottom line numbers are,
1oz x3 slices of Harvarti Cheese, $1.20
4oz 4 slices of 99% Fat-Free Ham, $1.25
E=410
F=240
Na=1330 >1g – remember to have 6-8oz of water later
CHO=0
f=0
s=0
Prot=152
T=392
0 61 39

Again. No carbs. Do you see how no carbs and low carbs just gets to be too boring after a while, and then people go back to eating ham-and-cheese bagels?

The NCD Ham & Cheese Bagel™

You didn't think I'd leave out bagels did you! Not by a longshot. We're not done being bad! We are going to be bad again later.

Chances are your energy will start to slide in two hours, so we have our 3sq 10g of 85% chocolate for a pick-me-up.

NCD Ham Harvarti & Choc™
E=473
F=285
Na=1333
CHO=15
f=4
s=8
Prot=156
T=456

If you go back to the first page of this chapter you will see our havarti cheese has E=110 calories per slice and T=104, the total calories are a little off. The T for 1oz of cheese is usually 108. This food label is a bit inaccurate. If the protein on the nutrition facts had said 7g instead of 6g, then the protein would be 4 calories higher and T would be 108 instead of 104.

This is why our E=473 and our T=456 are a bit of a discrepancy. Did you notice the ham? E was 20 and T was 20. So, let's just assume it's 473 calories and an approximately 500-calorie meal.

Our macros using T are, 3 63 34.
The fiber is only 4 calories so we are not going to crunch this with the net carbs.

It's a Lowcarb Nocarb meal, 3% carbs 63% fat 34% protein.

Again, no more than one of these ProFat or proFat meal substitutions per day, unless your calorie intake is 3000 per day, in which case you have the option of doing MWF 40 30 30 x4 plus 2 p/ProFat meals, and TRSaSu 40 30 30 x5 plus 1 p/ProFat meal.

But eventually once the fat is off, you don't need any p/ProFat meals. You lost all your visible fat and so your low-carb days are over! Hurrah! You can be bad again! Just eat 40 30 30 for all your meals, close the kitchen at 6-7-8pm, and snack on some cucumber sticks, snap peas, or cherry tomatoes later on if you need to (see ABC NCD Free-Vegetable Protocol™, page 315).

NCD Basic Carb Tweaking™
40 30 30 plus one p/ProFat = carb-tweak down
40 30 30 all meals
40 30 30 plus one "fruit meal" = carb-tweak up

When you control the numbers, you control the desired result.

CHAPTER 32

NCD Broccoli Soup™

The NCD soup recipes are a 6th Fat Cutting Tool. A 250-calorie soup snack FEELS like a 500-calorie meal. Thus, if you are eating 500 calories every 3 hours, totaling 2500 a day, you can substitute a soup for one of your meals and come in at 2250 for the day, 250 calories under.

However, ordinary soup recipes and store-bought soups won't do it. They're not 40 30 30. NCD soups are. The macros are the key.

You will need three different items. This recipe is a place where you can use leftover chicken, like how we did with the NCD BBQ Chx & PB Choc. We made 6 lbs of chicken breast, used half for the Orange Chicken, and used the leftover chicken to make BBQ Chicken Peanut Butter Chocolate. I like to make six when I do this recipe, but you could make just one, or any number that you want.

1. cream of broccoli soup
2. chicken
3. broccoli

1. Campbell's Cream of Broccoli
Food Maxx market, 10.75oz 305g can, buy 6 cans. Soup has doubled in price so buy it on sale or at a low-price supermarket, otherwise you'll be paying $2.99 a can at certain supermarkets. On sale you can purchase this at Food Maxx for $1.49.

Ingredients: water, broccoli, wheat flour, vegetable oil (corn, cottonseed, canola and/or soybean), onions, cream, CONTAINS LESS THAN 2% OF THE FOLLOWING!!!, salt, modified food starch, sugar, dried whey, soy protein concentrate, SPICE, SPICE EXTRACT, zinc chloride added to maintain vegetable color.

So you can see a few NCD questionables and red flags. But, it will taste amazing and so satisfying when we're done. Note, that the food manufacturer's "Go-To" oils are always the same bad ones.

NCD Refined GMO Oils™
1. REFINED GMO Corn oil
2. REFINED GMO Cotton plant seed oil
3. REFINED GMO Canola rape seed oil
4. REFINED GMO Soybean oil

How they get bottles and bottles of oil out of seeds is beyond me. I will tell you though that it takes A LOT of REFINING to do so. By the time they, press it, extract it, degum it, dry it, bleach it, and deodorize it, you're doomed. And as you will notice, all four are genetically spliced with cross-species DNA. Not good.

Add to that that they all come in clear bottles made of plastic, and you can quickly see that these are Poisons, or at the very least, Health Damaging Oils. Contrast this with olives. You squish out the oil, historically performed using a concrete wheel, and the oil is collected without heat, bleach, or chemicals, and bottled in glass that's amber in color to protect the oil from light.

NCD Oil Challenge™
Ask your order taker at the fastfood outlet what oil they use to fry in. Then ask them how often it's discarded and replaced.

They will say one of these, corn, cottonseed, canola, or soybean. When they tell you how often it's discarded and replaced, repeat it back, say, "Discarded every day?" They will likely be lying. Some lie some don't, many just look at you dumbfounded, as no one ever asks these questions. My point here is, they may drain it through a filter and reuse it, and refer to this as "changing" it every day. Then at the end of the WEEK, they discard it and use fresh oil.

NCD Double-Poison Oils™
1. Man Made – because it's genetically modified and very refined
2. Burnt – the color is not light yellow, it's dark brown black

And don't forget about DONUTS. A pathologist once brought a box of Krispy Kreme donuts to the lab to show appreciation, but sadly this doctor was ignorant of the facts, nutrition facts, and ingredients. The ENTIRE side of the box was used to list the ingredients. I think I counted 59 ingredients.

If it was me, I would have labeled it, Sugar Sugar and Burnt GMO Refined Vegetable Oil, not donuts. And put a big poison sign on it.

Our culture portrays eating these donuts as "fun and a well-deserved treat". Then, go spend $300 to see your favorite sports team play, and have a few drinks while you're at it.

Do you see how Hypnotized we all are?

We Fail To Think About What We Are Really Doing.
And how we are spending our free time.

Now it's socializing.

"Let's just keep them busy SOCIALIZING and they'll never finish reading that book, or even contemplate reading one."

I know many people, and this includes people with college degrees, who have never read a book since their early twenties. So the question is: What have they been doing? How have they been spending their free time over the past 20-30 years?

All that time is lost. They probably couldn't even tell you what they did. You my friend, can most-likely see what a waste of time it was. They never grew. They never learnt anything of value.

Our can of soup says 1/2cup 120mL, servings about 2.5, E=80 F=25 Na=750 CHO=12g Prot=2g. Campbell's keeps changing their nutrition facts. Bad Campbell's. And some stores have different labels for the same Cream of Broccoli soup. Try to find one that matches this.

You will notice that the nutrition facts are by volume and the front label is given in weight, Bad Campbell's. The can is 10.75 net weight ounces 305 grams. The nutrition facts say ½ a cup 120 milliliters mL. We can't crunch this because it's two-different types of measurements. Grrr. So, place a half-cup measuring cup on the scale and press "on", (zero it). Now, add soup to the half cup and place it back on the scale. I got 128 grams per half cup. And the entire can was truly 305 grams. So, 305g divided by 128g equals 2.38. There are 2.38 half-cup servings per can. Or, you can just use their "servings" number, which says "about 2.5" and multiply the nutrition facts by 2.5. So, E=80x2.5=200 F=25x2.5 =63 Na=1875 CHO=120 f=10 s=30 Prot=20 T=203, 59 31 10. This soup is 59% carbs 31% fat 10% protein. Our fat is fine at 31% but we need more protein!

2. Chicken Breast – to the rescue!
Boiled, Sliced & Diced, same as before. You will need 2oz raw 1.5oz cooked. E=60 F=5 Na=38 Prot=52 T=57.

3. Organic Broccoli Florets
TJs brand, 12oz 340g $2.29. You will use 4oz of broccoli per serving, so one bag provides 3 servings. We will buy 2 bags for 6 servings. You could also buy broccoli from the produce section and wash it in HOT water. Here's how I do it. Fill a big bowl, or a rinsed and towel-wiped sink, with hot water. Cut your broccoli heads so that the florets land in the water. When you are done, take your hands and wash them, like how you would wash a sweater or a sweatshirt in the sink. Lots of arm action. Pour the bowl of water and broccoli into a colander and let it drip a few minutes.

This is why I like washing my produce in a bowl. I have five different-sized bowls for whatever amount of vegetables I am washing. If I am doing 3 bags of snap peas, I use the second largest bowl, the "#4" bowl.

Since you need a "System" for washing your produce, so that it's fast and easy, and so that it works for getting them clean and pesticide-free, I recommend purchasing the follow bowl set.

NCD Kitchen Bowls™
#1 Small – 3⅞ x 9⅞ about 4x10 (inches)
#2 Medium – 4.75 x 11.75 about 5x12
#3 Large – 5.5 x 13.5
#4 XLarge – 6.25 x 15.75
#5 XXLarge – 7 x 17.5

The numbers are outside measurements; outside height, and outer-edge to outer-edge across the top. The bowls are made of hard plastic, so no soft plastic, but I am always on the lookout for glass bowls of the same big size, but they are impossible to find.

I actually prefer plastic for food prep because it's lightweight, just don't cook or store food in plastic. The XXL #5 bowl in glass would likely weigh 25 pounds, so that's probably why they don't make big glass bowls.

These are flat-bottom bowls with nearly vertical sides, not rounded sides. I have a colander inside each of the bowls that fits the bowl, so I call them the, #1 colander, #2 colander, #3 colander, #4 colander, and #5 colander. You will have to shop around to find these, but set them up as you will use them EVERY day, and you need five sizes for different-sized jobs.

You might think this is unnecessary, but when I've visited people and helped out in the kitchen, I found it a bit irritating because they only had two or three different bowl sizes. And then they wonder why they don't like to cook and would rather eat out.

NCD Food Prep Rule™
If it's not user-friendly, you won't do it.

Part of making your own meals means having a user-friendly system in your kitchen. So, it's a three-step goal.

Goal = Make All Your Own Meals
1. acquire the tools and set them up in your kitchen
2. have a system, a procedure, a series of food-prep steps to follow
3. then just do it – plan it, buy it, prep it, eat it

The NCD says you have to make your own meals, with the recipes to assist you, if you want to take control of your weight by taking control of the numbers.

Just like the ABC Water, you set it up once, and that's it. You're done. Just set-it-up and use it.

So, we have our six cans of soup, our two bags of 12oz organic broccoli florets, and our sliced-and-diced chicken, time to make some soup!

Step 1
Add the two bags of broccoli to a bowl of hot water and "Hand Wash" for 30 seconds. Transfer to a colander and let drip, then aliquot the broccoli into six medium pyrex bowls, 4oz each, eyeball it. Place the six bowls of broccoli on a shelf in the refrigerator, don't stack them. Now, place a can of soup on top of each bowl. Next, transfer 9oz of the cooked chicken to a 12oz sks jar with screw cap. You will remove 1.5oz with each serving.

Step 2 – Meal Time
Take one of your bowls of broccoli, the can of soup, and the jar of chicken. Add 2.0oz of water to the bowl of broccoli and microwave it two minutes. Pull the lid on the can of soup to open it and spoon the soup into the bowl and mix-and-mash it with the hot broccoli and water. Place the bowl on the scale and add 1.5oz of chicken, mix, put the remaining chicken back in the fridge. Microwave your bowl of soup one minute. This is warm. If you want hot, add another 30 seconds. Sprinkle with finely-ground black pepper, or fresh-ground pepper from a pepper mill, Enjoy!

You can also have 3 with black pepper and 3 without, for variety. It's good without black pepper as well. The broccoli calories are free (we will count its cost though), so our final numbers are:

E=260
F=68
Na=1913
CHO=120 nCHO=110
f=10
s=30
Prot=72
T=260 T-f=250
46 26 28 or 44 27 29

So our protein percent is key, it's 28 or 29%, good. Our carbs are 46 or 44%, but it's fine, and our fat of 26 or 27% is fine as well. It's very satisfying. No sleepy-brain or post-meal lethargy, on the contrary, it's a good "steady energy" meal. Plus you get a green, an estrogen-lowering testosterone-raising Green!

If you don't have cooked chicken breast available, you can buy 98% fat-free cooked chicken breast in a package. Trader Joe's "Just Caesar Chicken" is 3oz 85g E=110 F=10 CHO=3g Prot=21g, and I use this if I don't have cooked chicken breast prepared.

Carnation has a homemade Cream of Broccoli soup recipe, but it looks like a two-hour job. Or you could make a big batch of it and use half and freeze half for another time. One thing about Campbell's, their soups do have good flavor.

$3.12 per serving, if you get the soup on sale then it's $2.62, and if you buy nonorganic broccoli in the produce section for $0.99/lb then it becomes $2.05 per serving.

The low price of these recipes should motivate you further into setting up a system in your kitchen and making your own meals. Just take a step each week. Twelve months from now you'll be amazed when you look back.

CHAPTER 33

NCD French Onion Soup™

So your breadsticks should be stale. Remember the eight slices of leftover bread from the My Favorite Breakfast, and we sliced them in a stack in thirds, and placed them into a plastic container in the refrigerator. Well, we are going to use some of them next.

You will need 4 different items. You can make 4 servings, but we are going to make 8. Trust me, you won't be done eating them after just 4. This is sooo good. In addition to being a scientist, researcher, dancer-teacher-choreographer, I also worked as a cook, waiter, and bartender, and I worked at a supermarket. So, science, food, and body health and fitness, that's my expertise.

1. Organic French Onion Soup
Lassen's healthfood store, Pacific Natural Foods brand, 32floz 1qt 946mL carton, $4.99, buy 2. Filtered water, organic sautéed onion base (organic onions, organic dried onion, salt, organic butter, organic yeast extract, natural flavor), organic evaporated cane juice, organic onion flavor (contains organic sunflower oil), sea salt, organic garlic powder, autolyzed yeast extract, xanthan gum.

Not what we would expect from an organic product. But soups are notorious for having undesirables. The "organic sautéed onion base" says organic organic organic, and then natural flavor. Hm. Also, it lists "organic onion flavor" and then it just says "contains organic sunflower oil", but what else is in that onion flavor?

You could make your own from scratch, but it's another two-hour job. So, we'll use this. NF 1cup 8oz 240mL E=30 F=10 Na=720 CHO=5gx4=20cal f=0 s=3gx4=12cal Prot=1gx4=4cal T=34. We will use 1/4th the container, 8oz 1cup, per serving.

2. Spanish/Yellow Onion

Organic or not organic is fine as we are going to remove the outer peel. Buy two pounds. A 2lb bag of organic yellow onions costs $1.99 at TJs. Free calories.

3. Four Breadsticks

This means you will use one and 1/3rd slices of bread. This was our sprouted rye bread, F=10 per slice. We are going to use the fat-free sprout bread for this recipe. The numbers are about the same, but I usually make these breadsticks with the fat-free sprouted bread, and the 8 slices of rye from the My Favorite Breakfast are used for my next batch of 12 MFBs (4 loaves of bread = 5 batches).

TJs Sprouted Flourless Whole Wheat Berry Bread, 24oz 680g 20 slices $3.49. One slice 34g E=80 F=0 CHO=15g Prot=5g. Try to find one like this. Four breadsticks = 1⅓ slices, E=107 F=0 Na=215 CHO=80 f=11 s=11 Prot=27 T=107. This bread is 75% carbs 0% fat 25% protein. Ingredients: sprouted organic whole wheat berries, wheat gluten, organic dates, fresh yeast, sea salt, organic raisins, soy lecithin (emulsifier), cultured wheat.

Check this out. On the front label is says, "Glycemic Index 5.0 when tested on diabetics, Glycemic Load 0.9."

What do you think of that?

Information.

This company is informed. They understand GLYCEMIC LOAD. No mention of it being "low in saturated fat" and "low in cholesterol". Because why?

This bread company, and the Number Crunch Diet, pays attention to the important parameters, and we don't get distracted by the mainstream's blah-blah-blahs.

We know that the mainstream's broadcasting of information is not the full-100% truth. It may be that that's just all they know, and so that's what they broadcast. HOWEVER, they were broadcasting glycemic index ten years ago, but since then, it has gradually faded away. Much like how our wave blender has disappeared from the shelves. "Get rid of it, it's affecting our business."

JPM's information is like that. It is information, that, if applied, could have an effect on certain industries over time, a potential downsizing of the disease-treatment model, aka, healthcare.

But instead, we see sickness and ailments growing, and more and more hospitals, clinics, and therapies.

If everyone in America read and applied ABC NCD and made homemade meals from TCY, then in 2-5 years we would see standard healthcare and alternative healthcare getting smaller instead of expanding.

That's powerful.

That's why JPM books cost more. There's power in them. In that, you can shift control of your health from whoever controls it now, to taking control of it yourself – SELFCARE Healthcare.

If you haven't already done so, read my blog page on the website abcwaterandthenumbercrunchdiet.com, and read the part about where I refer to my brother-in-law's mother who lived to be 98 and never in her life went to a doctor for a problem, because – She Didn't Have Any.

This should be your goal as well. This is my goal for you.

4. String Mozzarella Cheese, Partly Skim
TJs or Safeway, TJs brand or Precious brand, 12 sticks or 24 sticks,

12oz 340g or 24oz 680g, you will need 12 sticks, 1½ per serving. Use the remainder for a ProFat snack, 3 sticks = 240cal ~250, 5% carbs 56% fat 40% protein. Or have 2 sticks and the 3sq 10g of 85% dark chocolate. I'll be using the TJs 12oz 12 sticks for $3.49.

Ingredients, milk, salt, enzymes, one stick 28g E=80 F=45. For 1½ sticks, E=120 F=68 Na=270 CHO=6 f=0 s=0 Prot=8gx4x1.5=48 T=122. Because this cheese is made from nonfat milk and regular milk, its percent fat is lower, 56%, instead of the usual ~75% fat of regular cheese, this makes its percent protein higher, 39.3%, nice. The minerals have a double-digit number, calcium 20% of RDV per serving. The RDV for calcium is 1000mg per day, so 20% is 200mg of calcium in one 80-calorie stick of this cheese. Amazing. We will be having 1½ sticks per serving, so 300mg of calcium.

Thank you dairy cows. They did all the work.

They did all the work so that you and I could have all the benefits, and get our 1000mg of calcium a day, plus magnesium and others.

NCD 3 Calcium Foods™
1. milk
2. cheese
3. yogurt

These are the Big 3. All other foods contain less, or a lot less, or they are fortified, like calcium-fortified orange juice and soy milk. If they fortify a product with something, then that "something" must be something we need to be getting in our diets.

NCD Fortified Rule™
Rather than eat fortified foods, eat milk and milk products that contain calcium naturally, and choose sprouted grains or true whole grains rather than refined-and-enriched bread products.

NCD Common Sense Rule™
Get some and use it!

CHAPTER 34

Pro-Discernment

JPM never touches on the political, nor are we anti-mainstream or anti-medical system. We are however, Pro-Discernment. That means, we look at it and decide from our Internal Divine what's really the situation.

Earlier I mentioned that the fastfood outlets raised the prices of their combo meals by $1+, the new normal being higher prices for food and a three-tiered system, where high-quality groceries are going to cost you more than average brands. Today, I purchased milk at the 7-Eleven, because I am going to use it in the NCD Tapioca Pudding™, and since it is going to be heated, I am not going to use raw milk. Well, when I said to the clerk, "You raised your prices," he said "Everything in the store went up." Wow. "Some things by 40%" he said. Double Wow.

In the 1990s, prices were stable for the entire decade. Gas was $1 a gallon, plus minus. Then in the year 2000 a new decade began, and a new Millennium, the start of a new 1000 years towards the next millennium in the year 3000. Not all generations experience this throughout history, this change of a millennium. If you were born in the year 2000, then the new millennium is all you've lived in. If you passed away in the 1990s, then all you knew was from the 20th century. So here we are 15 years into the new millennium and we've seen a steady increase in prices. While at the same time smaller packages and cans. One year the prices go up, the next year they make the packages smaller.

Making meals requires three things.
1. selecting your supermarkets
2. selecting your food items
3. exchanging your money for the items

The NCD encourages you to get the most nutrition for your dollar, and to not purchase foods with bad ingredients or with 90% profit margins. Spending is Voting. And this is one area in life that you have complete control over.

At the same time that inflation is occurring, wages and incomes for the middle class have been flat or going down in a lot of sectors. However, we have minimum wage becoming $15 an hour in Seattle. So I ask you this. When the president says he wants to help middle-class Americans, who is he referring to? The low-income poor and the corporate elite? For 25 years I've seen this pattern play out. The pushing down of the middle class. Meanwhile, China and India's middle classes are growing exponentially.

No point in fighting it, you'll just drive yourself to exhaustion. But you can DISCERN what's going on around you, and tell others.

If everyone "wakes up" and starts looking around, paying attention, then the lies of society will become mainstream.

If the information in ABC NCD, this book, and others, was to become common knowledge, the control would shift more into your hands.

Inflation is a dirty trick. They give you a pay raise, then they take it away with inflation.

So, within a year, all of these prices and meal costs are going to seem very outdate. So keep that in mind. The prices are meant to give you an idea. Not to be exact.

Step 1 – the onion
To make our French Onion Soup we are going to cut off the ends of the onions and remove one layer. Cut each onion in half and V-slice the onion into a large skillet. Cover and cook until soft. You don't need oil to cook vegetables, just cover and cook, the water in the vegetables will create a wet sauna-like environment. Perfect.

Step 2 – the soup
Mix the two quarts of onion soup and aliquot them into eight 16oz sks jars. Open the first carton and pour it into 4 jars, then open the second quart and pour it into the other 4 jars, just eyeball the levels.

Step 3
Add the soft-cooked onion to each of the 8 jars of soup. Cap & Refrigerate. Place your container of breadsticks and your 12 cheese sticks next to the soup so that it's all together in one place.

Step 4 – Preparation
Take one of your jars of soup, two cheese sticks, and 4 breadsticks, microwave the soup 1:00 and pour it into a ceramic coffee cup, break the breadsticks in half and place them on top, then shred one-and-a-half sticks of the mozzarella cheese on top. Pull the plastic up over the end of the remaining half cheese stick and put it back in the refrigerator. You can also break the cheese apart with your fingers and layer it on top. It won't be as nice, but it's faster and then you don't have to wash the grater. Because the cheese has a lot of protein, it's fairly easy to break apart, hence the name "string-y" cheese. But for your first batch, grate it, so that you have a perfect thick even layer of cheese on top. If you don't do it correctly, because you've never done it before, your broken-apart cheese pieces might sink to the bottom. You want to create a base with the breadsticks and then place the light shreds of cheese on top. My mouth is watering just thinking about this.

Step 5 – Baking
Place your coffee cup of FOS on the top rack of your toaster oven, or oven, and "Bake" at 350°F for 15 minutes, set a timer. (177°C)

Your cup should be about an inch or two away from the heating element, but off to the side from it, not directly underneath it. The other way is to use a four-inch wide ceramic ramekin and bake it in the ramekin if you want to eat your soup from a bowl.

When the timer goes off, use an oven mitt to remove your soup, it's hot, so be careful. Place it on a saucer, you can put a doily on the saucer if you are serving this to a guest, and place a spoon on the side. See website for photo.

Tip. Get the cheese to be light-to-medium brown on top, and you will feel like you are having the time of your life!

$2.16 per serving
E= 257
F=78
Na=1205
CHO=106 nCHO=95
f=11
s=23
Prot=79
T=263 T-f=252
40 30 30
No point in crunching it with the net carbs and fiber subtracted as it's not significant. It's perfect as is. And it feels perfect.

Soups have sodium, that's sort of why we like to eat them. Don't worry about the 1205mg in this one, or the 1913mg in the cream of broccoli. You are only going to have this one time per day. I include the sodium just for awareness of it, but it's really not an issue. What is an issue is Natural Flavoring, secret Spices, and other chemicals. I will continue to include it for awareness, meaning that, if you haven't had any water you will likely need a glass of water if the sodium is 1250-2000. That's all I'm going to say about sodium. Remember, good sodium is needed by your body. A little more sodium here, a little less there, it all balances out at the end of the day. And if you don't need it, you'll excrete it.

CHAPTER 35

CCC Pre-Counted Meals™

This chapter is going to cover the various macros that you will end up with if you tweak up from 40 30 30, for the person who wants to gain weight and muscle, and if you tweak down from 40 30 30, for the person who wants to cut fat.

So to start with, this may sound obvious but, if you eat all your meals and snacks as 40 30 30, then your macros at the end of the day are 40% carbs 30% fat 30% protein.

End-of-the-Day Percent Macros = 40 30 30
1750 calories a day = 3 meals and 1 snack of 40 30 30
2000 calories a day = 4 meals of 40 30 30
2000 calories a day = 3 meals and 2 snacks of 40 30 30
2250 calories a day = 4 meals + 1 snack of 40 30 30
2500 calories a day = 5 meals of 40 30 30
2500 calories a day = 1 meal + 2 D-meals of 40 30 30
2500 calories a day = 3 meals + 1 D-meal of 40 30 30
2750 calories a day = 5 meals + 1 snack of 40 30 30
2750 calories a day = 3 meals + 1 snack + 1 D-meal of 40 30 30
3000 calories a day = 6 meals of 40 30 30
3000 calories a day = 4 meals + 1 D-meal of 40 30 30
3000 calories a day = 2 meals + 2 D-meals of 40 30 30
3000 calories a day = 3 Double-meals of 40 30 30

Counting Calories made easy by Counting Pre-Counted Meals.

If this person wants a carb day on Sunday, or one day a week, and does the Fat Free Sunday, they can refuel their body's muscles with energy for Monday and for their following week of workouts. If you work out MWF, then Sunday you could do the FFS.

This day is best done by consuming fruit and fat-free protein. Because fruit doesn't sustain you for very long, it's best to eat every 2-2.5 hours, as in the following example.

06:00 up
06:30 fruit 250cal
09:00 fruit 250cal
11:30 fruit 250cal + 250cal of Fat-Free Protein
14:00 fruit 250cal
16:30 fruit 250cal + 250cal of fat-free protein
19:00 fruit 250cal
21:30 fruit 250cal + 250cal of fat-free protein (optional)
22:00 lights out

The fruit comes to 1750 calories and the FFP totals 500 calories, or 750 calories with the option.

Your first choice for fat-free protein is to take lean chicken breast, (F=0 or F=5 or F=10 at the most, not F=25 or F=30), and grill it on a double-sided grill. Slice it and eat it. It tastes excellent hot-off the grill. But there's a trick to getting it to cook evenly.

Chicken breast is thick at one end and thin at the other, and so the thin end gets cooked, and gets overcooked, while the thick end is still not cooked all the way to the middle. So, you can buy "Thin Sliced Chicken Breast" from Foster Farms, or you can make them thin yourself.

NCD Chicken Flattening™ technique
I had a heavy wooden cutting board that broke down the middle. Huh, I was upset about that, but it turned out to be a blessing in disguise. I ended up with two boards. One is 18-inches long 8-inches wide and 1-inch thick, and the other is 18-inches long 4.25-inches wide and 1-inch thick. I place the wider one on a low table,

place a chicken breast on it, and while holding the other board at the ends, I place it on top of the chicken breast and push down hard and flatten it. Perfect. It only takes a couple of minutes to flatten 8 chicken breasts and you end up with all your chicken breasts being ½ an inch thick. You heard it here first. *Food Network*, call me.

I used to buy the Foster Farms Thin Breasts but I have switched to buying the regular breasts for 50%-less money and just flattening it myself.

When you grill this flattened chicken breast, you will not need any seasoning or sauce, it will taste delicious hot-off the grill. Just place it on your cutting board and slice it in strips from end to end. The flattening also tenderizes it, so the chicken just melts in your mouth. For some "kick" shake a few drops of tabasco on top, mm!

Again, be sure your chicken breast is lean as we are not removing the fat droplets by boiling it, as we did earlier. Check the nutrition facts on the back and if it says E=140 F=30 put it back. It should say E=120 F=10. It is possible to find chicken that says F=5 and F=0. Albertson's sells "Chicken Breast Steaks" and the E=110 and the F is zero. But the standard one is E=120 F=10, and this is fine.

Now recall that boiled chicken weighs 3/4ths of what raw chicken weighs. Our NCD Boiled-Chicken Conversion™ is 0.75. For grilled chicken and skillet chicken it's 0.85.

NCD Grilled-Chicken Conversion™
Raw to Cooked = times 0.85
Cooked to Raw = divide by 0.85

This is why boiled chicken breast is a bit bland, it's lost a lot of its moisture and juices from being boiled in the water. But that's also how we get rid of the fat and the salt solution. Boiled chicken is ideal for when you need to "up" the protein of a dish, like how we did with the orange chicken and the broccoli soup. The mandarin sauce and the soup are the flavor components, so we just "upped" the protein with boiled "fat-free" chicken breast.

Our NF for chicken breast is E=120 F=10 Prot=26gx4=104cal T=114. If we multiply it by 2.2, we have E=264 F=22 Prot=229 T=251, ~250 calories. So, 4oz raw times 2.2 = 8.8oz raw, times 0.85 = 7.5oz cooked. We will serve ourselves a 7.5oz serving of cooked grilled chicken breast. The Na is 143, + 35 for 1t tabasco.

If you are lifting weights MWF your body will naturally gravitate towards chicken. Mine does. My DI wants chicken for my muscles after a workout. And a lot of chicken.

You will never get bored of this grilled chicken, but if you do, add the tabasco, or the buffalo tabasco, or a sprinkle of curry, or a little BBQ sauce, or Heinz 57 sauce. But go easy on the sauces, as we've already seen what's in BBQ sauce, and Heinz 57 sauce has high-fructose corn syrup last time I checked.

So if we have the 7.5oz of cooked grilled chicken twice along with our 1750 calories of fruit, that's 2250 calories. Our macros are 1750/2250x100=78% carbs, 22x2/2250x100=2% fat, and 229x2/2250x100=20% protein 78 2 20, or basically, 80 0 20.

NCD Fat Free Sunday™
Fresh Fruit and Grilled Chicken Breast

In addition to naturally gravitating towards chicken after a 45-minute weightlifting workout, I also gravitate towards fruit for carbohydrate replenishment. This is true for many people as well. They will be following someone's advice to get in shape, work out and eat a low-carb diet, but then they ask, "Can I eat fruit?" You can't really eat fruit on a low-carb diet. But if you work out, your body wants fruit afterwards. The NCD One Fruit Meal™ is ideal for this lifestyle. The 40 30 30 meals give you plenty of focused energy for your work out. Then afterwards, you have the One Fruit Meal to replenish muscle glycogen. What you do Post workout is more important than what you do Pre workout.

Now, if you had another serving of grilled chicken near bedtime, then your calorie total would be 2500, and your macros would be

1750/2500x100=70% carbs, 1.8% fat, 27.5% protein. This is the way I usually do it. Fruit results in an empty stomach, you won't sleep well on an empty stomach. This also raises my percent protein to 28% rounded, closer to the 30% daily target that I like to stay at if I'm working out. In grams, it would be 229cals of protein x3 chicken "meals" = 687 calories of protein ÷4=172 grams of protein for the day. You can get all complicated with the various protein-requirement formulas, grams per lean muscle mass blah blah blah, but that's just the fitness industry and advisors trying to "wow" you. The standard protein-requirement rule for someone working out MWF is one gram per body weight. So if you weigh 172 pounds, you should target your daily-protein intake to be 172g.

Also consider that fruit has some protein in it. If we use 5% protein as the average amount of protein in fruit, then our 1750 calories of fruit becomes 1663 calories of carbs and 88 calories of protein, rounded. So now our protein for this day becomes 229x3=687+88=775 calories, ÷4=194g of protein, and 775/2500 x100=31% for our daily protein percent. Basically, 70 0 30, 70% carbs fruit, 0% fat, 30% protein. A perfect carb-load day.

You can do FFS and FF Saturday, but it will get a bit boring to do this 2 days in a row. You really only need one carb-load day to get you pumped up again, back on your feet, and feeling charged and energetic. The other option is to do a Half Day of this carb-load.
06:00 up
06:30 fruit 250cal
09:00 fruit 250cal
11:30 fruit 250cal
14:00 fruit 250cal + 250cal grilled chicken breast
17:00 40 30 30 500cal
20:00 40 30 30 500cal
22:00 lights out

Total calories are 2250. Macros are 1000+200+200/2250x100= 62% carbs, 22+150+150/2250x100=14% fat, 229+150+150/2250 x100=23.5% protein, 62 14 24. These macros are, higher carbs, good protein, and lower fat. This would be good for a runner. But also good for the bodybuilder who wants to keep his muscles 100% fueled every day. When we take into account that the fruit has 5% protein, the macros become basically 60 15 25. Good protein, lower fat, and more fuel. You could do this every day, or alternate days, MWF half-day carb-load, TRSaSu all 40 30 30. Expect muscle growth if you lift weights.

If you added a second 250 calories of protein at 06:30, say 250 calories of fat-free turkey breast, or 50/50 fat-free ham and fat-free turkey, or fat-free ham fat-free turkey and scrambled egg whites with some tabasco or ketchup or curry, then you would be having 2500 calories a day and your macros would be 1400/2500x100 =56% carbs, 322/2500x100=13% fat, 229+150+150+~250/2500 x100=31% protein, 56 13 31. You can have tuna or fat-free fish, I just find it hard to eat fish plain. Assuming that your fat-free turkey, ham, tuna, or fish has a little fat in it, the macros would be basically, 55 15 30.

So this would give you 5%-more protein and 5%-less carbohydrates. This would be good for someone doing HEAVY weightlifting, lots of protein at 30-31%, a good amount of carbs for recovery and energy at 55-56%, and low fat, but not zero fat. You need fat too, so don't drop your fat below this 13-15%.

So as you can see, it's all numbers. And if you don't get them right, you won't feel right. You won't have the energy. If you overdo it with the energy loading, then you'll gain fat. This is so KEY if you are going to do a sport, plan to compete, or just trying to obtain a hottie body. Without this complete control of the numbers, your chance of attaining your goal is hit-or-miss. If you are a 20-year-old male, then you'll probably do it, if you are anyone else, you're going to have to use the numbers to get you there.

Chapter Endnote
Foster Farms 6-pack of Individually-Wrapped Chicken Breasts are usually about 8.8oz raw (7.5oz grilled, T=251). So, have 2 (or 3) on your FFS. They are also fairly thin, and flat.

CHAPTER 36

NCD Carb Tweaking™

If we do the one ProFat meal substitution, then we will have lower carbs at the end of the day. Your macros with the peanuts substitution would be,
CHO=200+200+200+23=623cal (using the peanuts nCHO)
Fat=150+150+150+396=846cal
Prot=150+150+150+91=541cal
Total calories = 623+846+541 = 2010cal (using the peanuts T-f)
623/2010x100=31% carbs, 846/2010x100=42% fat, 541/2010x100 =27% protein, 31 42 27.

By substituting one 40 30 30 meal with one peanuts meal, we basically just switch the 40 and the 30 on the carbs and fat. So instead of four meals a day of 40 30 30, with the one peanuts substitution we finish the day with our macros at about 30 40 30, 31 42 27.

This is a great way to cut carbs. And as stated earlier, don't substitute more than one meal per day. If you are a woman and you require 2250 or 2350 calories a day, eat four meals a day, 3x 40 30 30 and one peanuts. Add some calorie-free vegetables to carry you to your next meal if you feel low energy, or use the 1-2-3 squares of 85% dark chocolate, or the 1oz strong coffee and 3oz whole milk from ABC NCD. The free-3oz grapefruit works great for an immediate energy lift as it's sugar, but only 29 calories, 33 - 4 fiber =29nCHO. So remember, 3oz ~30cal, the NCD Free Grapefruit™.

183

It's just enough to boost your blood-glucose level back up into the normal range, without spiking it, and then you're fine for an hour until it's time to eat your next meal.

I hope you are getting a sense for how this "Eating Often" every 2-4 hours makes perfect sense, never going 5-6 hours without eating.

Your blood-glucose normal range is 70-110 mg/dL. Many people believe you should stay below 100. Think of it like this.

NCD Blood-Glucose Range & Flags™
Target = 80 +/– 10
Range = 70-90
Yellow Flag = 90s
Red Flag = 100s

The new rule for pre-diabetes diagnosis is a blood glucose of 125 or higher on two-separate occasions. So if you go to take a physical and they test your blood for blood sugar, if it's 125 or above and they ask you to have it drawn again in a week and it's 125 or above again, you are labeled Pre-Diabetic.

I agree with this. The medical system isn't always off-base. Some things yes, but some things no. In this case, they are really cracking down on diabetes and making the diagnostic criteria tough. But if you are walking around with your blood sugar in the one-hundreds, then it won't be long before you are a full diabetic.

So visualize your blood sugar as a highway lane, or a traffic lane.

120 – one step away from pre-diabetes
110 – too high
100s – red flag
90s – yellow flag ---
80 Target – stay between the lines 80 80 80 80 80 80
70 – lower end ---
60s – starting to notice a slowdown in energy and activity
50s – lower energy, some dull thinking, slight brain fog

For those of you up in Canada, your medical system has already got you thinking about blood-glucose range, and they gave it to you in a nice catchy phrase, "Six to Eight Feelin' Great". Your testing method is different than the one used in the United States. But, you understand that 8 is the upper limit and 6 is the lower limit, so 7 is your target, plus or minus one. Too high moves you towards type-2 diabetes and all of its related diseases, including body fat, and too low means you would rather sit than move and your brain would rather "veg" than read or think.

Aside. Type-2 diabetes used to also go by the name "Adult Onset" diabetes. But now, overweight children have it, so they had to drop the adult onset and just call it type-2.

If you are a parent and this is your child, I consider this to be child abuse. You are not looking out for your child and he or she is too little to know the effects of candy and sugar and too many calories.

And yes, the food manufacturers are to blame as well, but they will always throw it back on the consumer and say, "We didn't make them buy it."

Let's crunch our macros using 2500 calories a day, 4 meals of 40 30 30 and one peanuts.

CHO=200+200+200+200+23=823cal
Fat=150+150+150+150+396=996cal
Prot=150+150+150+150+91=691cal
Total calories = 500+500+500+500+510=2510cal
Macros are 823/2510x100=33% carbs, 996/2510x100–40% fat, 691/2510x100=27.5% protein, 33 40 27½. Again, a reversing of the fats and carbs from 40 30 to 30 40, while keeping our protein at close to 30%.

Let's do this substitution using our Guacamole-Tuna 3sq-Dark-Chocolate meal, as the protein in that one was closer to 150cal and 30%. Your turn. You crunch the numbers and then we'll see if we both match. It's good for you!!

185

Macros for a 2000-calorie a day diet, 3x 40 30 30 meals and one GTC ProFat substitution = 31.0 39.2 29.8, 31 39 30. Nice.

If we use the Ham-Havarti Chocolate meal, our macros are 31.4 37.6 31.0, 31 38 31. Still nice.

Again, we just reversed the carb and fat macros.

If we eat 2500 calories a day, 4x 40 30 30 and 1x ProFat, we have 32.8 37.3 29.8 or 33 37 30, (using the nCHO and T-f for the GuacTunaChoc meal). For the HamHavChoc meal we get 33.1 36.0 30.8 or 33 36 31, essentially the same.

When you begin to number-crunch design your own meals, just focus on where you are getting your protein from, and keep it at close to 30%. Then, 40% carbs for steady energy, 30% carbs for cutting body fat, 50-60% carbs, (the one fruit-meal substitution or HFFS), for bodybuilding and muscle gains, and 70-80% carbs, full-day FFS, to restock your muscles with fuel once a week.

NCD Carb Tweaking™
1. 30 40 30 Lower Carb – 1 peanuts or ProFat substitution
2. 40 30 30 Target – steady energy, no food cravings
3. 50 25 25 One Fruit Meal substitution, page 187 ABC NCD
4. 55 15 30 Half-day Fat Free Sunday with 2 prot meals 500cal
5. 60 15 25 Half-day Fat Free Sunday with 1 prot meal 250cal
6. 70   0 30 Full-day Fat Free Sunday with 3 prot meals 750cal
7. 80   0 20 Full-day Fat Free Sunday with 2 prot meals 500cal

Tweak down the carbs for fat cutting.
Tweak up the carbs for weight gain, muscle building, and sports.

The one fruit meal from ABC NCD page 187 actually crunched to 52 24 24, but there's some protein in fruit, so when we add that in it becomes 25-26% protein and 50-51% carbs, so basically, 50 25 25. They say grapes have 10 calories of fat, but that's from the oil in the seeds. Most people don't eat the seeds. Most grapes don't even come with seeds. Oranges have lots of fiber and that slows down the sugar, but mangos, pineapples and bananas, the tropical fruits, have only 6-13% fiber, so they are faster sugars.

NCD 40 30 30 Meal-Macros Variability Guidelines™
1-3% is not an issue
41 29 30 or 42 28 30 or 43 28 29 or 43 27 30 are all fine
4% is still fine
44 26 30 or 44 25 31 or 44 28 28 are all still fine
5% is about the limit
45 27 28 or 45 26 29 or 45 25 30 this is all still fine

We have to look at the entire meal, along with the macros. Also, we pay attention to how the meal makes us feel afterwards – the real reason for eating – how does it make you feel afterwards. Productive, or Sleepy. Perky and Fun, or Lethargic.

People eat for a FEELing of gratification. But on the NCD we eat for a feeling of ENERGY, sustained energy, 80 +/– 10 energy.

A 10% jump in carbs is a "Fuel Gear" change. A 10% jump down to 30% carbs is a lower fuel gear, so you will have to tap into your body fat for fuel. A 10% jump up in carbs to 50% is a higher fuel gear, more fuel available for your muscles to use during sports and exercise. And 60% is another gear higher, and 70% is another, and 80% carbs is the highest gear. If you use these "Gears" wisely, methodically, strategically, they will work for you, in tandem with your workouts, to assist you in achieving your fitness goals.

So, with control of the numbers, you have a huge advantage.

Diet Isn't Half The Battle – It's The Whole Battle™

Chapter Endnote – regarding page 184 ("never going 5-6 hours")
Intermittent Fasting is a valid technique, and you can experiment with this on your own. For example, eat a large 1500-calorie meal once a day, say at 3pm, then for breakfast the next day have a 500-calorie dessert, (fruit). So, you eat one meal and one dessert every day, 2000 calories a day.

CHAPTER 37

NCD Back Door™

In the main book, we often referred to "fixing the underlying problem" and by doing so your other problems should go away as a byproduct of "fixing the underlying problem".

I say that twice because it really translates to the ROOT CAUSE.

The medical and alternative-health industries would like you to believe that their product or treatment is going to help your condition, and it may some, but you have to get to the Root Cause.

If they did, however, they would go out of business. So they sort of just poke at your problem from the front.™

The *ABC Water and the Number Crunch Diet* goes in from behind, through the backdoor to get at your problem.™

This just means, we attack the underlying problems, and we keep attacking the underlying problems, until, one day, you wake up and say to yourself, "my problem's gone" or "my face looks younger" or "I can do backflips off a chair!"

While on vacation, we were heading to the lake to jump off the old railway bridge. My 15-year-old nephew said to me, "We should do backflips off the bridge." I said to him, "I was just thinking the same thing." It's about 15-feet above the water and we did backflips several times off that bridge. I was 45 then.

Being fit and looking good earns the respect of others. And the opposite is true. If you look like you're your age or older and you have a hard time taking part in activities at parties or family gatherings because your body is not up to the task, well, you are missing out. This book can help you shine and be a role model for your children, and the neighbor kids. They will respect that, as will your spouse, as well as your coworkers, clients, and your boss.

Take Delta Burke for example, or Christie Alley, celebrities that in the beginning looked great! Delta Burke was a beauty-pageant winner. These celebrity women became household names because of their beauty, charm, and appeal.

No one in the industry said a bad word about them. Untouchable.

Fast-forward, they gain weight. Delta Burke is told to lose weight or she may lose her spot on the sitcom *Designing Women* and Christie Alley is on the front of every supermarket checkstand magazine in a bathing suit. Now they're "Touchable".

By touchable, I mean, people are now being mean and hateful to them. Even cruel. Poor Christie Alley.

I once served Delta Burke and her husband "Major Dad" at the restaurant where I worked in Beverly Hills. Forgive me Delta for sharing this, but she had a large cheddar skins and a 32oz iced tea. If you don't know how cheddars skins are made, they are potatoes with the insides scooped out, then deep fried in a fat fryer, then covered in cheddar cheese and baked in the oven, and then you dip them in sour cream and scallions. A plate of five is at least 1500 calories. And 1000 of that is fat. Oh, I forget the bacon bits! They sprinkle bacon bits all over the melted cheddar cheese.

I'm not sure I could turn that into a 40 30 30 meal.

Had these beautiful women followed the Number Crunch Diet,

they could have taken control of their weight by taking control of the numbers they were eating.

All that to say this. When you look good, people leave you alone.

I mean, people don't mess with you. There's no cruelty, no snide remarks, no dirty looks, no rude attitudes. No fat pictures.

You're RESPECTED.

We live in a visual world, and everyone is judged on looks. I've seen many women who are fifty or more pounds overweight who dress to-the-nines at their job in order to get some respect. If they would just fix the weight problem, that respect would be there.

The posture book that I plan to write will refer to a client I had back in my dancing days. She was a mess. Educated, but over-weight and bad posture. I fixed her posture and she went from a size 13 to a size 2 dress size. During one of the dance classes, I was working with her and I commented on how much she had improved. When I put my hands around her waist, they touched. She was a true size two. By the end of the season, she was a completely-different person. Outgoing, confident, throwing dinner parties, and she had even become the life of the party, taking the stage away from her competitors. At the end of two years, she had been promoted at her job to as high as a woman could go, the people above her were "key" men, the kind that only get replaced by other men. She wore mid-length dresses that hung straight down, her narrow waist, high heels. She looked like a million bucks. And she was 45. She looked better at 45 than she did at 35.

This woman took my help and ran with it. She gave me the credit for her promotions and transformation, but I was just doing my job as a dance teacher. Her husband was fat and lazy. He worked 7-to-4, and watched TV all evening, every evening. He became fearful of losing her because now she was way out of his league.

So I ask you. Which person would you rather be?

That question ends in a question mark. Those are the questions that I want you to answer. The other questions that don't end in a question mark, those are to make you think and ponder.

Well, I know the answer. YOU WANT TO BE THAT WOMAN!

So start thinking about posture. It's a component of fat loss. As is alkalinity.   One person recently told me he lost 30 pounds by drinking alkaline water. It makes perfect sense.

By drinking alkaline water you perform a full body detox, the fat falls off and you have less fatigue so your energy goes up so you need less calories and the fat falls of some more. It's a vicious cycle. But a good vicious cycle.™

So by going in through the backdoor, by fixing your nutrition, your calorie intake, and your poor food choices, the fat comes off.

When the fat comes off, your hormones fall into place. As a byproduct.

By going in through the backdoor, we fix your body's hormonal balance. Hormonal Regulation.

As a byproduct of being on the NCD, your hormones become regulated. They will naturally fall into place.

Recall Chapter 44, G Load, glycemic load, page 188 ABC NCD. If insulin, (your blood-sugar hormone), ain't happy, all of your other hormones won't be happy either. If insulin is up down round and round, so too will be your thyroid, your pituitary, your adrenals, your thalamus, hypothalamus, and all the hormones that these areas secrete and regulate.

The other "experts" will treat each of these areas of your body in a sequence. They'll start with X, and if that doesn't work, they go after Y, and if Y doesn't fix it, they'll try Z, and on-and-on. At a certain point, they may tell you they've exhausted all options and thank you for coming.

More accurately, they should say, "Thank you for playing." The game. Of life. We led you to believe in us, and you did, and now we have your money, and you have the learning experience from it.

My job is to protect you from that. And it's everywhere. And more and more every day. Oh, "Our new formula does yada yada yada." Or, "Our new facility has state of the art…" yaaawn.

Don't be fooled by all that. It's hypnotism. Listen to the inner you.

Your symptoms are signs of compensation for something you are doing wrong.

Health problems are caused from a lack of Something Good that you weren't doing, or Something Bad that you were doing, or a bit of both, a combination of the two.

Don't forget, a "symptom" doesn't have to be "back pain" or "joint pain". A symptom can be something as small as, forgetting how to spell a word, or using a calculator for addition because you forget how to add, or your vision for seeing things far away isn't sharp like it once was, or your skin has lines that weren't there before, or your voice is weaker and you have to clear your throat before you speak. Pay attention to these small signs. As they lead to bigger signs down the road.

The day that you notice a gray hair or a gray whisker, aging has begun. Stop. Ask yourself, what things am I doing that are Bad, and what things could I be doing that are Good. Ponder that.

So the Number Crunch Diet tackles hormonal imbalances by going through the backdoor, by fixing the underlying problems.

The Root Cause.

CHAPTER 38

NCD Skillet Chicken & CC™

Okay. We are going to do the skillet chicken and carrot cake so you can see how you can have dessert but not gain weight because the carbfats in the dessert are built into the meal. I hope we have time to do the cheesecake one. Oh, and the chocolate mayonnaise cake. That one is pure heaven. And it's so simple to make. Easy to make, but not easy to bake, because if you undercook it it turns into chocolate mayonnaise fudge cake! And we can't have that. Actually, we can!

But we are going to begin with the skillet chicken because you don't get to eat the carbfats until you've eaten your protein. And you better have your side of snap peas, green and yellow bell peppers, green beans or beets, now, as this meal doesn't have a vegetable. We just did broccoli and onion, so now it's time to be bad again!

But seriously. If you have read this book up to this point, then you deserve a reward, and for those of you that read *ABC Water and the Number Crunch Diet*, and this book, you are my people. My hat is off to you. This is the only diet that gives you complete nutrition, with maximum freedom, combined with total control. It's not easy but it pays off. Since the mainstream is closed off to material like this, I ask for your help with word-of-mouth advertising. Grassroots. I've got lots more recipes, self-health protocols, and the posture book is something I've wanted to write for 30 years.

This recipe makes 10 and requires 3 different items.

1. chicken breast
2. coating – flour, salt and pepper
3. carrot cake

1. Chicken Breast

We will need 5.3oz of raw chicken breast times 10 meals = 53oz or 3.3 pounds, plus a few ounces for waste that gets trimmed off, so 3.5 pounds of raw lean chicken breast. If you see visible fat anywhere, you can assume they are hiding additional fat underneath the breasts, in which case, buy 3.7 pounds. Again, I buy the 6-pound size and use the leftover chicken for something else. Generally, you will trim off and discard 1oz per pound.

For those of you who are wondering if we are ever going to eat any of the other parts of the chicken besides the breasts, the answer is yes! NCD Drumsticks & Pudding™, two onion-coated baked chicken drumsticks with rice pudding for dessert, have a vegetable 30-60 minutes prior as a before-meal snack. NCD Teriyaki Chicken™, white and dark meat chicken with egg noodles, teriyaki sauce, coleslaw, and six! squares 20g of 85% dark chocolate, that's $1/5^{th}$ of the bar. So it's not always fruit for dessert.

4oz 113g of raw chicken E=120 F=10 Prot=26g. If we use 5.3oz then we end up with E=159 F=13 Na=86 Prot=138 T=151. Again, all we see is 91% protein, a little fat, and a little sodium. No chicken breast that says "up to 15% solution".

NCD Chicken Pumping™

Ideally 1% solution. 3% solution maximum. No 15% pumped up chicken breast.

Since you are reading the Calories and Fat Cal on the nutrition facts label, then once you're done, drop you're gaze down to the Sodium and make sure it's not 470!

One last thing about chicken-breast numbers and that is, sometimes you will see nice looking breasts on sale and the E=140 and F=30. Smart and Final's chicken is like this.   When I boil it there are almost no fat droplets, so in this case, although it says F=30, it's really more like F=10 or 5 or 0.   But this is with regard to boiling. For this recipe we are using a skillet, so no fat will be drawn out of the chicken, therefore, use one that's F=10.

2. NCD Skillet Chicken Coating™
This recipe is actually taken from a restaurant in a rather touristy hotel.   It's flour, seasoned salt, and black pepper, (FSP).   But you need the right ratios.

Flour.   King Arthur brand, whole wheat flour.   One ingredient, unbleached 100% hard red whole wheat flour.   1/4c 30g E=110 F=5 CHO=21gx4=84 f=4gx4=16 s=1g=4 Prot=4gx4=16 T=105.   Is this a whole grain?   What's the percent fiber?   16/105x100=15%. Double-Digit percent fiber!   Yay!   I think we've found a whole grain!   No B vitamins and iron added back in, that's another clue to a whole grain.   On the front they brag, "100% of the wheat germ and bran" and "Never Bleached Never Bromated".   That just sounds nasty doesn't it?   There is bromine in some orange soft drinks, and in Mountain Dew, (Brominated Vegetable Oil).   In my 2000-page eight-pound clinical-chemistry textbook, with the chapters tabbed, color coded, highlighted, and notes in the margins, it lists bromide underneath chloride underneath fluoride.   King Author is proud of the fact that they don't use it in their flour. They also say on the front "100% committed to quality".   I like that.   This whole-wheat flour is so finely ground that it could pass for enriched white flour.   I use it for baking as well and it's perfect.

For the amount of coating, we will estimate 6 grams of flour per serving, E=22 F=1 Na=0 CHO=17 f=3 s=1 Prot=3 T=21.   (We are sprinkling 9g, but we lose about a third to the skillet surface.)

Black Pepper.   Use finely ground.   It works better than regular or coarse.

Salt.   Sea salt, Celtic salt, Real salt, Kosher salt, Himalayan salt, just not white refined iodized aluminum-ized tablesalt. Look for one that brags about being unrefined and contains trace minerals.

If you want more "kick" in the flavor, the original recipe uses Lawry's Seasoned Salt. Ingredients, salt, sugar, spices (including paprika, turmeric), onion, cornstarch, garlic, tricalcium phosphate (prevents caking), natural flavor, paprika oleoresin (for color). So we have a double red flag, spices and natural flavor.

I have switched to using sea salt, but the Lawry's seasoned salt does make it taste more like Kentucky fried chicken. Proceed with caution. If you find yourself getting hooked on this skillet chicken, then it is this product that's doing it. See ABC NCD for the NCD Quitting Plan™ two step chemical addiction program, page 177.

Lawry's seasoned salt used to have monosodium glutamate in it, and some versions of it still do, so buy one that says "contains no MSG" on the front. Apparently, that MSG stuff is bad for you ;)

There are no calories, but it says on the nutrition facts label that $1/4^{th}$ tsp 1.2g has a sodium of 380mg. Does that seem like A LOT of sodium to you, or is it just me? If we crunch that into grams, then 1g÷1.2g=0.833x380mg=317mg. ONE GRAM of Seasoned Salt has 317mg OF SODIUM. We are using 32 grams of this product to make our seasoning, so that's 317x32=10,144mg of sodium. The batch divides into 20 (use half and save half for next time), so we are looking at ~500mg of sodium per serving. One-tenth of the carrot cake has 223mg of sodium, so our total sodium is ~723mg. We're fine. Except for that natural flavor.

Step 1 – the FSP coating (10 servings x2)
Place a 16oz sks jar on the scale, zero it. Add 180g of flour. Press tare or zero. Add 17g of black pepper. Press tare. Add 32g of seasoned salt. Cap & Shake. For you measuring-spoon people, it's 1¼ cups of flour, 2T pepper, 2T salt (Lawry's or sea salt, or 50/50).

Someone told me they didn't know what "tare" meant. I said, you don't have a kitchen scale do you? Tare sets the scale to zero. It's written on all three of my scales. Yes, I have 3 kitchen scales.

Step 2 – the chicken
Place your trimmed and flattened chicken breasts in the skillet. Sprinkle them with the FSP coating, turn them over and sprinkle again. Add one cup of water to the skillet, cover and cook at 350°, set a timer. At 6 minutes, flip them over and replace the cover, cooking 6 more minutes. Unplug the skillet at 12 minutes, remove the cover and proceed to slice the chicken into strips on a cutting board. Aliquot into ten 12oz sks jars 4.7oz of chicken each.

Our 5.3oz of raw chicken x 0.85 is 4.5oz cooked, plus 0.2oz for the coating, so 4.7oz.

Use the sks jars with screw caps and the chicken will last 10 days.

Step 3 – the carrot cake
TJs carrot cake, freezer aisle, 23oz 652g, $5.99. Sugar, carrots, soybean oil, enriched bleached flour (wheat flour, malted barley flour, niacin, iron, thiamine mononitrate, riboflavin, folic acid), eggs, walnuts, cream cheese (pasteurized milk and cream, cheese cultures, xanthan, carob and guar gum stabilizer), butter, baking soda, salt, cinnamon, pure vanilla extract, modified corn starch. Good. This tastes exactly like my mother's homemade carrot cake so why spend hours in the kitchen making it. You will know this has real cream cheese frosting when you eat it. Mmm!

1/8th cake 82g E=320 F=170 CHO=37g Prot=3g. Try to find one that matches this. We are having 1/10th E=255 F=135 Na=223 CHO–118 f–3 s–86 Prot–10 T–263, 51% fat 45% carbs 4% protein. It's fat and carbs with a tiny amount of protein. It's a CARBFAT! Dessert! But that's okay, because it's the carb fat portion of our meal. So don't feel guilty. I never do.

Open the box and remove the paper wrapped around the edge of the cake. Removing the paper wrapping is hard to do if the cake was thawed, so keep it in the freezer until you're ready to aliquot it. Cut it in half, equally. Now, cut each half into five wedges, that's 4 cuts. Place each triangle-wedge of cake in an extra-small pyrex bowl, times ten. Some of the slices will get a bit messed up, but that fine. Cover & Refrigerate.

The box says the cake is 652g, mine weighed 663g, close enough. Using their numbers we have 652÷10=65g. Each of your aliquots should be 65g. I eyeball it, but in the beginning you should weigh them. Place the xsmall bowl on the scale, add the wedge of cake, if it's 85g then remove some, if it's 54g then add some. You get it.

The frosting is the sugar part so be sure to divide that up evenly as well.

So, grab a plate, place your skillet chicken on it, you should have saved the 10th chicken aliquot for your current meal, and if you didn't have a vegetable earlier, then add one now on the side, say, carrot or cucumber sticks. Pray, change gears from working to eating, and sit down and enjoy.

If you are dieting, and trying to cut fat, then don't do this next part. But if you are on maintenance calories or you worked out yesterday or you're going to work out later today, then add 50 calories of fruit. Or you could have boiled chicken with 40g of BBQ sauce. Or, you could have two 3oz grapefruit later on. Or, you could have beets with this meal, on the side with the chicken, and have one 3oz grapefruit later on. Carbs are your fuel, so if you need them, have them. If you don't need them, then omit this part.

This meal is crunched with the 50 calories of fruit and it looks like this.
E=159+22+255+50=486
F=13+1+135=149
Na=86+500+223=809mg
CHO=0+17+118+50=185
f=0+3+3=6
s=0+1+86+50=137
Prot=138+3+10=151
T=151+21+263+50=485

Our macros are 38 31 31. We are not going to crunch this with the nCHO and fiber subtracted T-f because there are only 6 calories of fiber, and we are having dessert, so those 185-CHO calories are 185 real carb calories.

If you omit the 50 calories of fruit, then the sugar drops from 137 to 87. The NCD likes to keep "s" the sugar to less-than 100. We need some sugar, but if we go over 100, just be aware of it. One meal a day like this is fine. I am having this meal with the 50 calories of fruit and 137 calories of sugar because I did seated rows, shoulder press, deep leg squats, and tricep pressdowns earlier, so this meal with the fat, the chicken, and the 137 calories of sugar, is going to create an anabolic effect.

It happens every time.

An anabolic effect is what EVERY professional athlete lives for. And MANY of them have done so illegally.

I figured out how to create an anabolic effect with food.

You can drive a Hummer and live in a two-million-dollar home, but if you are standing in a room next to someone with a great body and a muscular physique, all of a sudden, you're not that popular. Same goes for you women. The hotter you look the better. Life just goes your way. Waiters will give you extra avocado on your salad for no charge, the clothing-store clerk will give you the sale price even though the sale ended last week, the auto shop will wash your car just for getting an oil change. You will be amazed at how much free stuff comes your way. And did I mention job promotions? A big chunk of that is based on visual.

When You Look Good And Feel Good – You Shine

That's really the life you want. Why settle for less.

CHAPTER 39

NCD Buttered Popcorn™

Yes! We are having popcorn. With Butter! How fun is that! But it's story time first. It relates to this recipe. And there's always a point at the end so play along.

I brought my buttered-popcorn skillet-chicken to work at the lab once, and well, once I melted that butter in the microwave and poured it on top of the popcorn, everybody in the lab came a running. I brought extra and made two more servings of the popcorn because I like to feed people. AND, because many women are so deprived of real food, so I would show them how they can eat and not feel guilty about gaining fat. One time my friend's 68-year-old mother told me she had been on a diet her entire life. How depressing.

So my coworker asked if she could take the buttered popcorn that I made extra home with her, absolutely I said. She was overtaken by that buttered popcorn and couldn't believe how good it was. What was really happening, the way I could see it, was that her Divine Inner Intelligence was saying "Ah, finally, butter nutrients and popcorn nutrients, I ran out of those two years ago."

I don't know what's in butter exactly or popcorn exactly either. That's my Divine Intelligence's area, that's his job. My job is to assist him with his job. The two yous remember. Inner you, Outer you. Think of eating for the inner you first, and the outer you second. But, you see, if you follow the mainstream worldly belief, you will never hear talk like this. They don't want you to listen to your inner Divine, they want you to listen to their divine. Your inner Divine is the big "G", and theirs is the decoy, the little "g".

The recipe makes 8, and you need the FSP chicken that we just made, a bag of organic popcorn, and one stick of organic butter.

1. Arrowhead Mills Organic Popcorn
Lassen's Healthfoods, 28oz 793g $5.99.   Ingredient, organic yellow popcorn. 1/4cup 46g E=170 F=20 CHO=33g f=7g Prot=5g, try to find one that matches that. 1/8th of the bag is 99 grams, but we lose 16% when we pop it due to unpopped kernels, so, 99 grams times an 84% yield = 83g, our serving is going to be 83g. E=307 F=36 Na=0 CHO=238 f=51 s=7 Prot=36 T=310.

Front cover bragging says "excellent source of fiber". And it sure is, 51/310x100=16.5% fiber. How many grams of fiber is 51cals?

2. Organic Butter, unsalted
TJs brand, 16oz 454g $4.99, pasteurized organic sweet cream (milk), lactic acid, 1T 14g E=100 F=100 SF=7gx9=63cal Na=0 CHO=0 Prot=0 T=100. This food is a satfat, 63% satfat. Saturated fats are animal fats, meat, cheese, dairy, butter, and our oddball plant, coconut oil. God put that oddball in there for a reason, so if you don't have coconut oil in your cupboard, go buy some and use it in baking. A stick of butter divides into 8 tablespoons, so we will have three-sticks remaining. You can make this again, that would leave two-sticks remaining for the curry sauce of the NCD Curry Chicken™, or you can vacuum seal the sticks and use them later on. I do this recipe twice and follow it with the curry chicken, so by the end, I've gotten butter out of my system, and popcorn.

You will look at movie-theater popcorn and feel nothing.

NCD Ultimate Butter Sensation™
Use RAW butter!
Raw milk butter, it has sooo much buttery flavor that by the end of

the week the butter is coming out of my pores and my skin smells like butter. But people like the smell of butter. It's like cocoa-butter lotion but more buttery and less perfume-y. Kidding!

Step 1 – the popcorn
Add 99g of popcorn kernels to the cup of the air popper, (place the cup on the scale, zero it, add kernels until it says 99g). Add them to your popper. Place the popper in the sink and place a cylindrical pale under the mouth of the popper. Plug it in and set your timer. At 1:45 minutes, place a two-foot-long paper towel over the pale and mouth area. At 2:00 the popcorn will be at the top. At 2:30 it's 90-percent popped. Unplug it at 3:00. Let it cool. Dump the popcorn from the pale into your #2 colander and then hand transfer the popcorn into a 3.5-quart plastic container with lid, K-Mart Martha-Stewart brand (may be discontinued).   Discard the unpopped kernels and repeat seven more times.

Tip. My air popper is the Presto Poplite, Walmart, $15, buy two. I kept burning out my popper because it would overheat halfway through my batch. So now I alternate. Use one popper, then let it cool off while you use the other popper. So, each popper has to pop 4 servings, rather than forcing one popper to pop all 8 servings. Now my poppers are ten years old and still going strong.

Tip. For your first round of popping, the popper is cold. Let it run 15 seconds. Turn it off. Add your kernels and turn it on. You will do this for servings 1 and 2 only. For servings 3-8 the popper will be warm when you start it, this way all your popping times are the same. If you start with a cold popper, then add one-extra minute to the first run.

When you are done, you should have 8 containers, each with 3.5 quarts, 14 cups, of popcorn. That's 28 half-cup handfuls!

Step 2 – the butter
Grab eight 2oz sks jars, cut the stick of butter in half, then cut the halves in half, then cut the quarters in half. That will leave you with 8 evenly-sized butters, 1T each. If you cut them like that, you

won't need to weigh them. Don't cut it from end to end, you most likely won't end up with equal portions.

Transfer them to the 2oz jars, Cap & Refrigerate.

Tip. Leave two butter servings out at room temperature, so that when you microwave it, it doesn't splatter, and it requires less heating time.

Yes, I am aware of what people say about microwaved water, that it changes the water into something foreign looking. But one minute, two minutes, three minutes, that's less time than it takes to boil water. And it's pretty hard these days not to use a microwave, they're everywhere. Just try to avoid cooking in one, 10-15-20 minutes. Although you can microwave a potato and have a hot "baked" potato in 5 minutes, (the NCD Soyaki Chicken & Baked Potato with sour cream and chopped green onion – mmm!).

Step 3 – the chicken

Cut and trim your raw chicken breasts, flatten them between two boards, cook them in the skillet with your FSP coating, and slice them up on your cutting board. You need 4oz raw x8 = 32oz or 2 pounds, plus 2oz for trimmed waste, so, buy 2.2 lbs. Your 4oz raw chicken is 3.4oz cooked, multiplied by the 0.85 raw-to-cooked conversion. Add 0.2 ounces for the coating for a total of 3.6oz of FSP Chicken. Aliquot them into 8oz sks jars for a 10-day shelf life in the refrigerator, thanks to those airtight screw caps!

A final word about popcorn. Women who are trying to cut calories sometimes make air-popped popcorn and keep a bowl of it on the table to snack on when they feel hungry. This is fine to do as it is filling thanks to all the puffed-up fiber, but keep in mind that it is corn carbs, not free carbs. Before you know it, you've finished that bowl of plain popcorn and had 120 calories of carbs. These extra carbs may slow down your fat-loss progress.

It would be better just to make this recipe meal, and then you won't want popcorn and you won't feel hungry.

Party Time! You can eat this meal in two parts, sit at the table and have the chicken with a vegetable, or without a vegetable if you had one earlier, then grab your buttered popcorn and sit on the sofa, read your book or plan your next recipe meal, or just stare off into the distance and ask, "What's it all about…Alfie."

Place your 2oz sks jar with butter in the microwave and nuke it on high for 15 seconds, then for another 15 seconds at 50% power. If you press "three zero start", it will splatter. So 15 high and 15 low.

Pour it on top of your popcorn, sprinkle it with sea salt, and enjoy.

See the photo at www.abcwaterandthenumbercrunchdiet.com

E=549
F=147
Na=? (~0.5g for the FSP coating) (plus your salted popcorn)
CHO=255 nCHO=201
f=54
s=8
Prot=143
T=545
T-f=491
The macros with the fiber subtracted = 41 30 29.

Eventually, I want to have a set of secret web pages with pictures of all the meals, along with additional information you won't find anywhere else, so be sure I have your email address so I can give you free access (keep your receipt to show you bought the book).

Chapter Endnote
Okay, you need a quick meal and you're away from home, what do you do? Burger King. No, I am not recommending this. It's just an option. Order one Whopper with Cheese, No mayo. Toss the top bun in the trash. You now have a roughly 500-calorie meal with about 104 calories of protein, about 108 calories of carbs, and about 310 calories of fat, 21 59 20. High fat, but low carb, with a reasonable amount of protein, for $4.83.

CHAPTER 40

The Wrap-up

Well, that's it. 200 pages for the follow-up books – Twelve Changes a Year, Volumes 1, 2 and 3. We'll continue on in the next volume, but start adding these to your life over the next 12 months so you can track your calories by counting pre-counted meals.

Start with the Flaxseed Shakes. They are the most important, nutritionally. When you start consuming freshly-ground flaxseed you will likely sense that you're deficient in omega-3. On your first swallow you'll say "Mm this tastes good." But not the mmm-flavor good, like in the hawaiian-pizza drippings, or the peanut butter and dark chocolate, but more like a, "Mmm good, this feels good." Your body will sense the nutrition and say "uh, mm, yeah, this feel good", "good for me". You're low in this essential fat that your body cannot make, and you can't really get it from foods as it's too unstable, so you eat those foods and you're still deficient.

Omega-3 is what a flax seed was made for. Then consume them fresh after grinding up the seeds, and then you've got them. You've got those unstable U-shaped fatty acids in your bloodstream and your DI will send them to wherever they need to go, brain, eyes, membranes, adrenals, men – to your man organ. Maybe you're losing it down there because you're short on omega-3. And vision. I said your skin would get softer over time, but what if your vision improves, your reading vision and your night vision. What if all that is omega-3 deficiency?

One person I spoke with who worked for an ophthalmologist told me that cataract surgery was a booming business because of people's lens becoming hard. Both omega-3 flax and fish fat DHA EPA are found in the same organs and tissues in the body, so don't forget that the other thing you need to be doing is the NCD CLO Shots™ (see Chapter 55 of ABC NCD).

If you didn't read *ABC Water and the Number Crunch Diet* then Welcome! and CONGRATULATIONS!, as reading this without the 350 pages of the main book would be very hard, I would think.

If you read ABC NCD then you likely got to the end and still had some questions. It is impossible to cover everything in one book. So, now you are on your way with 12 recipes over the next 12 months. We will fill in more of the gaps in volume two, along with more tips, and another sampling of recipes. We never got to the chicken caesar salad, or the chinese chicken salad, the german potato salad, the other soups, new england, chicken noodle, gumbo, the orange shake, the egg nog!, the chili dog, the burgers, double cheese, cheese and bacon, the poppyseed cake, the chocolate mayonnaise fudge cake, the chicken & cheesecake, the cherry cheesecake topping, the pecan "pie", all the beef recipes, fish tacos, more chicken recipes, the thanksgiving meals, more egg meals, more profat meals, oh!, and I haven't even started to give you the ProCarb meals, 150 calories of protein, no fat, and 350 calories of carbs, for the bodybuilder or athlete, oh!, and the Forgotten Protein Meal, oh man, we didn't get to that one.

Well, we will just have to gedder-all-done in the next volume.

See you there!

God Bless You!

Don't forget YouTube – public and private videos for Subscribers.

CHAPTER 41

Summary Index

Even though I've only read 94 books in the past 14 years, if I go back 30 years to my university days, then it's well over 100. The odd thing is, I Find Indexes To Be Completely Worthless. You go to look something up in the index and is says page 17, 49, 50, 178, 254. So you go to page 17 and it's one word, just the word, no definition or information. Then you go to the next one, page 49, you look and look, and it's just another use of the word, then to the next pages, and on and on. I gave up using indexes years ago. So, what I find more effective and useful is a Summary Index. Kind of like a full-book review.

I also like to "trademark" my work. Poor Nikola Tesla invented so many things, you can see dozens of pictures of his patents on the internet. Sadly most people don't know he even existed. Or those artists who wrote songs in the 1950s and sold them for a few hundred dollars, and the songs became top ten hits. We all recognize the song, but no one knows the person who wrote it.

Everything on the pages of this book is original, I created it, in my quest for answers and my quest for protocols for how to put those answers into action.

If I sound braggadocious, that's because this stuff really works! Try it. Take the journey. You'll see the changes. It's not packaged fancy, but good things often come wrapped in plain packaging. ☺

Let me tell you how Awesome! I think you are, as getting good nutrition and maintaining weight through calorie control are key answers to living a long and healthy life – and looking HYA!™

The Flaxseed Shake Recipe is my most amazing invention, because the U-shaped fatty acids of omega-3 need to be ground fresh.™

NCD Molasses Flaxseed Shake™ NCD Maple Flaxseed Shake™ NCD Honey Flaxseed Shake™

Insoluble fiber doesn't get absorbed, it stays within the colon, soluble fiber gets absorbed but it creates a gel that slows down the release of sugar.™

NCD Five Healthy Sugars™
1. Molasses – blackstrap
2. Maple Syrup – grade B
3. Honey – raw and unfiltered
4. Fruit
5. Cane Sugar – organic and minimally processed
And some organic stevia occasionally.

NCD Omega 3 Protocol™

I was tricked by this "one roll 71g" until I checked it. Therefore, verify the weight of your food items, especially bread products.™

Remember, you'll be miles ahead of the average person after a while, when it comes to health, selfcare, and NUMBERS!™

Flax seeds are 31% omega-3 fat!!!!!!! About one-third omega-3.™

Hemp seeds are loaded with minerals, good fats, and protein.™

So you have all the advice givers saying "eat more omega-3s", and now you are armed with everything you need to do it.™

JPM – from Advice to Results™

The advice givers also say "healthy fats", but they really have no idea what that means, or they are trying to sell you their product.™

NCD Edible Fats™
1. 3 6 9 plants
2. saturated animal fat and coconut oil
3. fish fat

I hope you can see the difference in the two types of food available for you to eat. God's way versus man's way.™

Pay attention to "purity", that's my advice.™

NCD Emergency Meal™

The all fruit-and-vegetable diet is the "Get Well" diet.™

By going on a vegan diet, you fix your acid-base balance.™

ALKALINE DEFICIENCY™ – the hidden aspect to your health.

Added salt and naturally-occurring salt are not the same.™

The devil is in the details, and the devil removed 90% of the minerals.™

If you see high potassium, you can assume it's unrefined and the minerals have not been removed.™

This shake could just as easily be called the NCD Mineral Shake.

Don't make the NCD Shake Mistake™ – follow the NCD Leafy Greens Protocol™ to get your leafy greens.

NCD Secret Ingredient™
LIQUEFIED Nonfat Cottage Cheese™

JPM – Your First Choice For Selfcare Strategies

You have to crunch the numbers to see what you are really eating, and paying for.™

Cheating never gets you anywhere, except back where you started, or worse.™

The NCD Flaxseed Shake™
1. NFCC – for lean protein
2. Unrefined sugar – for minerals and sweetness
3. Raw Milk – for protein, fat, carbs, minerals, and PROBIOTICS!
4. Flax Seeds – for omega-3 fat and other fats and fiber

Sugar Has A Function – Use It But Don't Abuse It™

Bottom line – It's not a meal. It's missing the 30% protein.™

You think you are eating healthy, but you are simply eating dessert.

Dietary Confusion™ – where you continually change what you eat.

Refining takes the minerals out. Unrefining leaves them in.™

Aliquot, Aliquoted, Aliquoting – the new terms in dieting.™

Rather than take steroids, eat eggs.™

NCD Dietary Fats Explained™ (in the main book explains it best).

With the NCD Omega 3 Protocol™ you should have no deficiency.

Use glass containers instead of plastic and become a Plastiphobe!

Do you remember the following from page 159 of the ABC NCD? That's exactly what's happening.™

NCD Hawaiian Pizza™ Woohoo!

Using a pita in place of pizza crust is a NCD original idea.™

Doctors are disease identifier and disease treaters. Here at JPM we focus on the ANSWERS.™

If you have inflammatory skin rashes, consider "things" living in your colon that are excreting toxins.™

Do the Parasite Cleanse, and stay on the maintenance protocol.™

The mainstream media has embraced Pollutants and Chemical Contaminants, but they have yet to discuss the other part.™

People should think twice about wearing flip flops when walking about in public places.™

NCD Whole Grain Rule™ – double-digit fiber percent.

They listed every single spice they use, no "Secret Spices".™

Let thy food be thy medicine and thy medicine be thy food.

NCD Bragging Features™
Be sure to read the label to see what they "Brag" about.™

Dessert doesn't always have to be cookies, cake, and ice cream.™

35 minutes divided by 6 = about 6 minutes per pizza. You have time for that.™

NCD Roasted Peppers Chicken Pasta™ – also 6 minutes/meal.

The NCD says, if you can find a good product then why make it from scratch.™

An overabundance of chemicals in your diet and lifestyle are going to show up somewhere in your body, sooner or later.™

Interesting that the organic zucchini was grown in Mexico and the nonorganic zucchini was grown here in the USA.™

Toss your Teflon-coated pans and skillet in the trash and switch to the new ceramic-coated nontoxic cookware.™

The minute you notice that the Teflon is peeling off – toss it!™

The NCD uses the Pyrex glass bowls and rectangles for food storage, along with the glass jars from sks-bottle.com.™

Forget that French al dente way of cooking noodles, cook them soft so that you don't have to work so hard to digest it, and to make those carbohydrates available now not later.™

Record your cook time, so that the next time you make a recipe you don't have to think about it, and food prep becomes faster.™

When cooking and meal prep becomes easy and mindless, you won't resist doing it. It will seem just like any other chore.™

NCD My Favorite Breakfast™ should become your "go-to" breakfast. And the variations will keep it interesting.

The NCD recipes don't contain Trans Fat.™

Just make your own meals yourself and stop consuming things that make you age and steal your health drip by drip.™

Fruits and vegetables that don't get peeled, like tomatoes, really need to be organic, as the pesticides get soaked into the surface.™

VOTE WITH YOUR DOLLARS – it's how you have the most say.

Make food choices based on your Internal, instead of your External, and your food choices will change.™

Peanut butter is not "high in protein", but you have to crunch the numbers to see it.™

This jam company is giving you a quality product for your money.

Choose Bolthouse Farms for pomegranate juice as it has nothing else added. Plus they give you "Information" about the product.™

Do you see how Nutrition is going to fill you up and satisfy you?™

You don't need to reinvent the wheel, the system is already invented for you. Just jump in and begin!™

Cook your food to 3/4ths doneness and allow it to finish cooking off heat to just right – NCD Off-Heat Cooking™.

NCD Breadsticks™

The black part on burnt toast is carcinogenic, as are the black grill marks on a hamburger patty, steak, or flame-broiled chicken™

You don't need to worry about cholesterol or saturated fat on the NCD, it's all within range.™

The next time someone says they're drinking red wine because it's good for you, suggest pomegranate juice and see what they say.™

NCD BBQ Chicken & Peanut Butter Chocolate™

The NCD allows you to have treats and desserts because the carbfat part is built into the meal. But you have to crunch the numbers to get it right. You can't just guess.™

Raw chicken in 1-3% solution has a sodium of 75mg on the nutrition facts. Chicken with 15% solution has six times that.™

Boiling lean chicken breast, F=10, removes the fat droplets and results in NCD Fat-Free Chicken™.

NCD Boiled-Chicken Conversions™
raw to cooked = x 0.75
cooked to raw = ÷ 0.75
For grilled or skillet chicken, use 0.85.

Natural Flavor is a code word.   The NCD doesn't $upport nondisclosure on a food label or within the ingredients list.™

Cocoa has theobromine, a slightly weaker version of caffeine.™

NCD Chicken Dicing Technique™ – and start with a sharp knife.

The person who worked out can benefit from the extra carbs, but if you are wanting to lose fat a bit faster, omit the fruit dessert part.™

40% carbs is a nice steady energy.™

When you cut your daily carb intake to 20 or 10%, your mind becomes fixated on food because your brain is short on fuel.™

Caffeine will allow you to keep going, but at some point it's all going to come crashing down like a house built with cards.™

You should feel completely satisfied and fine with 40 30 30 meals.

When you control the numbers, you control the desired result.™

Your goal should be that 100% of your food-budget money is spent on groceries from supermarkets.™

NCD Orange Chicken™

Be alert to the phrase "less than 2% of" in the ingredients list, as what usually follows are the chemicals you can't pronounce.™

NCD "Spice" Rule™
Spice, singular, strongly suspect MSG. Spices, plural, may just be spices or it may be spices and MSG.

Organic-Food Companies Disclose
Processed-Food Companies Hide

Would you trust your spouse if he or she was hiding things?

Food manufacturers can get around the MSG labeling by modifying it slightly and so now it's called something else.™

If you feel a "hook" or a "kick", suspect chemical flavoring.™

pH is hidden, hence, root causes are not found, just treated.™

Do you see how pH affects things?™

Understand the difference between percent fat or protein by weight and percent fat or protein by calories/energy.™

You canNOT make omega-3 fatty acids. You have to eat them.™

Omega-6 is also an essential fatty acid, but not a seek-out fat. We get omega-6 from fresh raw peanuts, hemp seeds, corn, sunflower seeds, and it's found in soybeans, all nuts, and other fatty foods.™

The NCD recipes contain omega-6, but it's omega-3 that is hard to get, and the proper way (fresh) (freshly ground).™

Rancid oil is right down there with burnt oil and man-made.™

NCD Food Prep Rule™ – Clean As You Go

NCD Salmon Mixed Vegetables Focaccia™
NCD Salmon Mixed Vegetables Egg Rolls™

Okay! Are you ready for some DHA and EPA!

It's not so much what it looks like, it's what's IN IT.™

But with the NCD you get both. It looks good and it's loaded with what your Divine Intelligence needs.™

If your lifestyle is "low activity", you can get by with 15% protein, because you have very little Muscle Turnover. But a healthy lifestyle includes exercise for the heart, lungs, muscles, and joints.

The NCD is not against other macro percents. If you just completed a heavy and intense weightlifting workout, a 40% protein meal is ideal and needed.™

With complete control of the numbers, you can work the plan in any direction you want.™

60% carbs + 30% fat + 10% protein is dessert, be alert to that.™

NCD 6th Method for Food Addiction – rename it, call it like it is.™

The person on that diet had better, drop their calorie intake, track their calories thoroughly, and close the kitchen at six.™

It's better to have extra protein than not enough, as your body can convert the extra protein to energy, but fats and carbs cannot convert to protein.™

So if you are going to be deficient in something, don't let it be proteins or essential fatty acids. NCD Dietary Essentials™ p233

Are they hiding anything? Nope. You could make it yourself. But why bother when this is essentially homemade.™

Bottom line, the carbs in this meal are wrapped up and slow. There is no insulin spike.™

See how they disclose what they are using for seasonings.™

Enriched bread products have the vitamins and minerals removed and then they add artificial versions back in.™ Backwards.

Buy a one-liter of cola at the minimart and see how much they are charging for it.™

You do have power over the food that's made. It's called money.™

Apparently, those plastic food containers that people have been using all these years weren't safe. Imagine that.™

The NCD meal titles can seem a bit nerdy, but that's because the goal is to have you get a picture of the meal. Chicken Tremendous tells you nothing. We also don't use words like Luscious, Juicy, Succulent, and Scrumptious, that the mainstream companies often use to appeal to your base nature.™

So all you'll hear are Amazing! Terrific! Awesome! and Mmm!

Food shouldn't be in your #1 spot. Nor in the #2 spot. Food's just food. Nutrition for your Divine Internals. But there's no harm in making it taste good and having some fun. And some bad!™

NCD Ingredients Rule™ – If it's not a food, it's a food additive.

The NCD focuses on the GOOD things, the POSITIVES, we should be doing, while merely being informed and aware of the bad, so we can make better choices.™

The reader can explore the bad on his-or-her own. Though, instinctively, you already know, or have a pretty good idea.™

I have never heard my Divine Intelligence ask for maltodextrin.™

"With a side of modified corn starch and some hydrolyzed soy protein." The same is true for your Divine Intelligence also.™

The NCD preferred dessert is fruit. Because if we eat fruit alone as a snack, it's 100% sugar, fine and good for the person working out, less fine for the person whose goal is to cut fat. Fruit makes up 50% of the phytonutrient plant color-pigment group, vegetables being the other 50%, so we can't just not eat fruit.™

Many people have lost weight just by stopping drinking sodas.™

They turn off the IV infusion of dextrose being pumped into their veins. Their insulin goes down and they stop storing food as fat.™

You just read the answer to body fat. You're keeping your blood sugar spiked with too many carbs.™

That IV of glucose has a lot of different names. Lattes, donuts?™

Glenn Beck joke. His wife asked, "Does this dress make me look fat?" Glenn replied, "No, your fat makes you look fat." Ouch!

When you take control of the numbers, you take control of your marriage.™

By keeping your protein steady, at 30%, you'll maintain steady energy and a stable mood.™

If you want to bolster your energy for the gym, do the NCD One Fruit Meal.™

Or, save the fruit for after the workout for a better pump.™

The two things my body asks for after a workout are, Chicken and Fruit. Good protein and plant sugar.™

Because the NCD is a Numbers-Based plan, you can use it to achieve any goal that you have, weight loss, weight maintenance, weight gain.™

The NCD is a holistic program. It considers the whole picture.™

The whole picture includes that of a Divine Source, an Inner Knowing, and we look to that to guide our choices and when deciding the truth about things.™ Discernment.

Without the truth you are a prisoner and a slave, and you don't even know it. Mass-media programming has got you.™

I was there once.

The NCD Foundational Principle™ – get the truth and get free.

And while you're looking for the truth around you, be sure to check in the mirror, that's where it all starts.™

DISCERNMENT – Use that word like a flashlight, to help you see.

You will quickly catch the attention of others, as the mainstream's modus operandi is to – Keep You From Discerning.™

JPM UNtruths™
1. Partials – missing part of the truth
2. Clouded – confused and wordy stories to conceal the truth
3. Partial Plus – truth with lies, SPIN, it seems believable
4a. No Truth – the person lying to you is fooled
4b. No Truth – the person lying to you knows the truth

I encourage you to "Man-up" and correct lies and liars in their tracks, because once they gain a foothold, you're done, your marriage, your kids, your country.

All of the wrongs you see in society today can be attributed to people in the past not standing for truth and allowing lies to roost.

Somewhere at the root of all problems is, a Lie.™

Switching from soft drinks to teas is like the drug addict switching from drugs to alcohol.™

JPM's goal is to have you miles ahead of the mainstream masses, not jumping from this to that to the next, going around in circles.™

NCD Franks & Relish™

Organic Organic Organic, don't you just love the sound of that word! The word itself says, "wholesome, natural, healthy and pure".™

The NCD says No! to colors and dyes. We eat yellow, red, and blue plants, not yellow, red, and blue dyes.™

The NCD Orange Shake™ and the NCD Chocolate Milk™ work great for the double-meal option.™

In today's society, everyone wants more ENERGY. But only occasionally do we hear in the mainstream the word CALORIES. But, calories are energy.™

And CALORIES are calculated from our THREE MACROS.™

Again, not something you'll hear too much about in the mainstream, just a little surface information.

Get your calories and your macros right and your energy will be there.™

Seriously, after a while, you've had so much fun eating that you are bored with food. It becomes, just food.™

Companies that sell food try to portray it as something it's not. Fun, romance, and celebrations, are about People and The Event.™

Never Forget INNOVATION – New and better ways.™

NCD Taco Salad™

Latte coffee companies are focused on margins and profit, not on value and nutrition.™

Vote for companies that sacrifice profit to give you value, and you'll be more likely to see more of these good companies in the future.™ The flipside of that is also true.

Say to a friend, "Oh, I don't waste my money on that, it's 90% profit margins and I get no nutrition in exchange." Be a Thinker!

Front label "bragging", No Preservatives, No Artificial Colors or Flavors. Hm. I starting to think those things are really bad for me. Good thing I'm paying attention.™

Two years from now, you'll be able to number-crunch design your own recipes!™

You can't just be looking HYA, you have to have a sharp mind too!

You have more calcium in your body than all of the other minerals combined. Where would we be without cows?™

So if you hear someone say, "beans are high in fiber", you can follow it up with, "Yes, and black beans are 29% fiber."

Many people eat carbs mindlessly, never understanding what a carb is for.™

But if you have body fat, you have energy sitting there waiting to be used.™

NCD Three "Starch" Categories™
1. sprouted bread, true whole grains, and occasional enriched
2. potatoes, peas, corn, sweet potatoes, yams, pumpkin, and beans
3. fruit, fresh, dried, juice, and the NCD Healthy Sugars™

Most other diets will tell you you can't have fruit, or very minimal, and only certain ones.™

The NCD is really the "All Your Dreams Come True!" diet.™

NCD One Fruit 'Meal'™
NCD One Nocarb 'Meal'™

All spices are antioxidants, but the yellow pigment of curcumin, found in turmeric, used in curry, is the Champion.™

There is power in plant colors.™ Phytonutrients.

NCD Spicy Rule™ – medium at most. Never spice to hot.

NCD Dip Washing™ – six submerges in hot water, flick, repeat.

The NCD recommends buying a Wave Blender.™

Cook the ground beef to MW, slight pink, then unplug the skillet and continue to mix-and-flip off heat until just right.™

NCD Off-Heat Cooking™

When making a meal recipe, take a look at the Pros & Cons. The pros will help you to see how "worth-it" your time and effort is.™

PubMed will never validate this, but the NCD Taco Salad, with its animal beef, the red tomatoes, the beans, raw cheese, and dark leafy green lettuce, creates an Anabolic Effect.™

I believe the numbers have a lot to do with it as well, 40 30 30 and 500 calories.™

Of course, you have to have lifted weights previously to feel the anabolism. If you want anabolism without lifting weights, then eat ten ounces of freshly grilled steak or oven-baked prime rib, "The Sirloin Steak Effect".™

NCD Peanuts™   NCD Chili Peanuts™

NCD ProFat Meal™ 10 60 30 and 500 calories.

Listen to your body.™

Lower carb is for getting lean, trimming down. If you want to expand and grow, lower carb is not the way to go.™

Don't get greedy with wanting the fat to come off. Just get the ball rolling, then stick to it and get busy with life.™

NCD Kitchen Closed At Five™ is still one of the best ways to wake up each morning thinner and leaner.™

proFat is a ProFat meal, but with ~20% protein, instead of 30%.

NCD Lowercarb Cycle™
Jan Feb – 8 weeks 40 30 30 x4 + one p/ProFat meal
Mar April May June – 40 30 30 x5
July Aug – 8 weeks 40 30 30 x4 + one p/ProFat meal
Sept Oct Nov Dec – 40 30 30 x5

Twice a year for 8 weeks your daily-carb percent will be ~30%, lowercarb. Then followed by 4 months of daily carbs at 40%, mild-to-moderate carbs.™

This is very methodical. You will not even notice you're dieting.™

Ladies, you may think that 2500 calories is too much, as those diet companies have you thinking you need 2200 calories a day. Put in a full 16-hour day, add the NCD Recalibration Exercise, cross-country-ski walking, 45 minutes a day, and space your meals out so that you close the kitchen at 3-hours before bed.™

If no walking, then do 40 30 30 x3 + one p/ProFat, 2000 per day.

NCD Fat Cutting Tools™
1. NCD Lowercarb Cycle – as above
2. NCD Kitchen Closed at Five, 3-4-5 hours before bed
3. Sporadically omit a portion of the carbs with any 40 30 30 meal
4. NCD Recalibration Exercise – for hormonal balancing
5. NCD Free Vegetables – see ABC NCD, NCD Grapefruit™

If you use these 5 tools, the fat will come off, and then melt off, and then you're there.™

The NCD – a Unique Approach to Weight Management™

Bridging the Reader from Advice to Results – JPM

But first, you have to control the numbers you're eating by tracking the number of pre-counted meals you eat each day.

NCD Tracking™ – to control it, you have to track it.

The NCD says, think of your body as a business.™

NCD Guac & Tuna™   NCD GuacTuna & Choc™

NCD fastfood restaurant option, there aren't very many, but it does help for when you're away from home and you have to eat something.™

The NCD says to read the information on the food product. Simply take two minutes to read the entire box or package and you'll be amazed at how much you'll learn, and how it adds up over time.™

And you'll become known as the Master of Food Trivia!™

Trivia for them, information and knowledge for you.™

The NCD encourages you to choose God's foods over man-made foods because – they resemble your bodyparts.™

The NCD Clear Colon™ – a full colon is a sluggish colon, and robs you of energy. Keep it light. Use the NCD Guac & Tuna if you find yourself needing a laxative.™

The key is to have everything you need for your meal all in one place.™

If it's not "Grab-&-Go" all in one place, you'll opt for something else that's easier.™

If someone opens your refrigerator door and wants to know why you have cans of tuna on the shelf next to your guacamole, refer them to amazon.com for a copy of this book!

You need to make your "Meal Making Mindless". Keeping it all in one place helps you to "Get-A-Visual" of the meal, and then with the visual, the next thing you will do is "Take-it & Make-it".™

NCD Pray Before Each Meal™ – to change your biological state.

The theobromine will give you energy and keep you in a good mood!™

NCD Lowercarb 8-Week Cycle of Meals™ (30 40 30)
13 days   Peanuts
 8 days   Guacamole-Tuna & Chocolate
13 days   Spicy Peanuts
10 days   Ham-Cheese Roll-ups & Chocolate
13 days   Peanuts

You can also do 4-Weeks Lowercarb, every third month.™

rBST, hm, doesn't sound to me like anything God made.™

It takes MUSCLE to burn calories. In fact, your calories are being burned by your MUSCLES. So use them. And the harder you use them the more calories you will burn.™

And Hard means Hard. Not Long, LBC – long boring cardio.™

NCD Fat Loss Alternative™
Stay on maintenance calories, just add weights and cardio. For the person who just can bear to eat less than they are now.

Intense exercise will make you hungry later on, so plan your exercise to end 30-45 minutes before your next meal.™

The preferred method for fat loss is to keep your calories the same, but add Cardio-Weights to your lifestyle.™ Fitness Transformation

Ham and Havarti ROLL-UPS! Two will be more cheesy than ham, and one will be more hammy than cheese.™

Do you see how nocarb and lowcarb just becomes too limited and boring after a while, and then people go back to eating ham-and-cheese bagels, or they "cheat" every fourth or fifth day.™

We're not done being bad!™

Not more than one ProFat or proFat meal substitution per day. Exception, if you are eating 3000 calories a day, you could do 40 30 30 x4, a peanuts, and a ham-cheese-choc, but don't do this more than every other day, 3x a week MWF, and then TRSaSu 40 30 30 x5 and a peanuts or ProFat, or TRSaSu 40 30 30 x6.™

Too few carbs and your energy drops. When your energy drops, your calorie burning drops. So you're no longer cutting fat.™

But eventually, once the fat is off, you don't need any profat meals. You've lost your visible body fat and so your lowercarb days are over. Hurrah! You can be bad again!™

NCD Broccoli Soup™   NCD French Onion Soup™

NCD 40 30 30 soups are a 6th Fat Cutting Tool, as the 250 calories feels and lasts like a 500-calorie meal.™

So you could substitute a NCD Soup for a meal and cut your daily total calories by 250 just with this 6th tool.™

Ordinary soups won't do it though. They're not 40 30 30. The macros are the key, and the total calories.™

NCD Refined GMO Oils™ – Corn, Cotton, Canola, Soybean.

These four are ubiquitous in the restaurant and fastfood industry.™

These four oils come from plants that have had their DNA changed, no longer God made plants, then the oil is Extracted, Degummed, Bleached, and Deodorized.™

A diet that includes these "Four-Horsemen-of-the-Apocalypse" oils, from deep-fried food, will have you looking YA, your age.™

NCD Double-Poison Oils™
1. Man Made Oil – used in fastfood and restaurant fryers
2. Burnt Oil – used in fastfood and restaurant fryers

Our culture says "donuts" are treats, fun, and something you should buy for a group of people to show your appreciation.™

As a NCD reader, you are aware. So you know that this is cultural deception for the benefit of others. You see right through it.™

In reality, donuts are, sugar, sugar, and burnt GMO refined oil.™
In case you missed that, the first sugar is the frosting, and the second sugar is the white flour, which is, chains of sugar.

Sometimes just eliminating the bad is all you need to do to get healthy and have more energy.™

SOCIALIZING is another cultural deception. Decades ago, people worked and were productive 12-14-16 hours a day. Socializing was only a small fraction of their day, and then some on Sunday.™

If you were 12, you were considered old enough to work. And you learned the value a dollar the hard way. By earning it yourself.™

Also back then, people aspired to become learned individuals. They valued books. And they read them. It was understood that you had to read books if you wanted to move up in life.™

What have many of today's people been doing in the past 10-20 years? How have most people been spending their free time? Are they utilizing their time? Or are they just squandering it?™

NCD Kitchen Bowls™ – 5 sizes for all your needs

NCD Food Prep™
Create a user-friendly system in your kitchen for food prep. Otherwise, you won't like to cook and you'll opt for eating out.

NCD GOAL = Make All Your Own Meals™
1. acquire the tools and set them up in your kitchen
2. have a system, a procedure, a series of food-prep steps
3. then just do it – Plan-it Buy-it Prep-it Eat-it

The NCD says you have to make your own meals, with the recipes to assist you, if you want to take control of your weight by taking control of the numbers.™

Just like the ABC Water, you set it up once, and that's it. You're done. Just set-it-up and use it.™

The low price of these recipe meals as compared to eating out should motivate you further into setting up a system and making your own meals at home.™

JPM – Our mission is to get, and keep, you looking Half Your Age.

Check this out. On the front label of this sprouted berry bread it says "Glycemic Index" and "Glycemic Load". What do you think of that?™

No mention of "low in saturated fat" or "low in cholesterol" because why? Those are "distracting parameters" that the mass media tries to sell people on. The NCD readers are informed readers and they know what's important.™

Like the $15 wave blender disappearing from the store shelves due to its innovative design being a threat to all other blenders, the information published by JPM is equally a threat to traditional ways of thinking about health and taking care of yourself.™

If traditional healthcare is so good, why are we seeing more and more people utilizing medical care? What's causing the ever-growing numbers of adults, and children, to be so unhealthy?™

JPM's publications cost more, because they're worth more.™

Allowing you to potentially shift the control of your health from whoever controls it now, to taking control of it yourself, Selfcare.

My brother is "his own dentist", as told to him by his dentist 33 years ago. My brother-in-law's 98-year-old mother never went to a doctor her whole life. What do these people know?

This should be your goal as well. It is my goal for you.

200mg of calcium in an 80-calorie stick of cheese. Thank you dairy cows. They did all the work.™

NCD 3 Calcium Foods™ Milk Cheese Yogurt

NCD Fortified Rule™
If something is fortified, then we need whatever it is that they are adding. Rather than eat fortified foods, eat the foods that naturally contain those vitamins and minerals.

NCD Common Sense Rule™
Common Sense seems to be becoming less-and-less common. Don't let that be you. Keep reading and it won't be!

JPM is not anti-mainstream or anti-medical. There are thousands and tens-of-thousands of people who would rather just take a pill or undergo a procedure, ignore their health issues, or, just suffer with an ailment until the end. JPM is pro-discernment.™

Pro-Discernment puts JPM at odds with the mass media, who, simply don't want you to discern the truth about things. If you believe in Jesus and satan, Truth and lies, then we encourage you to seek the truth and follow it. "I am the way, the truth, and the life:"

Meal-Making 3 Requirements™
1. selecting your supermarkets
2. selecting your food items
3. exchanging your money for the items

The NCD encourages you to get the most nutrition for your dollar.

Avoid buying items with bad ingredients and 90% profit margins.

Spending Money is Voting™

Prices for groceries continue to go up, and the prices of fastfood are going up also. Regardless of the actual price, the underlying premise is that you can eat far better food for 2-3 times less money by buying groceries rather than by eating out.™

Inflation is a dirty trick.™

Pay attention to what's going on. All the small inches add up.™

No need to add water or oil when cooking vegetables in a skillet. The moisture from the vegetables creates a wet sauna-like environment.™ Perfect

Get the cheese to be light-to-medium brown on top, and you will feel like you are having the time of your life!™

Soups have sodium, that's one reason why we like to eat them. That, and in addition to being filling, satisfying, and having half the calories of a regular meal.™

Stay tuned for the NCD Lunch Trios™
Small bowl of green salad, a cup of soup, and half a sandwich. A bit of work, but enormously satisfying.™

When you eat right, you naturally become happy after eating.™

Just like if you eat wrong, you become unhappy after eating.™

In the Greek language there are four words for the word "love", agape, eros, philia, storge. Keep this in mind when hearing words like salt, sodium, milk, etc. There are many types of salts, not just one. Good salt is good. You need a steady supply, especially if you perform Sweat Cardio or you tend to drink a lot of water.™

The NCD pays attention to only the "bad" salts, as listed on the ingredients label, and we try to limit our daily intake of bad salts.™

Counting Calories made easy by Counting Pre-Counted Meals™

FFS, Fat Free Sunday, can refuel you muscles for your next week of workouts.™

NCD Chicken Flattening™
Tenderizes the chicken breast and allows for even cooking.

Add a few drops of tabasco for "kick". It's made from 3 foods, vinegar, salt, red peppers. The Buffalo one has garlic.

Boiled lean chicken breast is great for when you need to "Up" the protein content of a meal.™

The standard protein requirement is 1g per pound of body weight. This is equal to 4 calories of protein per pound of body weight. If you ate 40 30 30 x5, then you've had 150x5=750 calories of protein, ÷4 = 187.5g or 188g of protein per day. You're covered.™

Better to have a bit more than a bit less when it comes to protein.™

It only takes one day of FFS to reload your muscles. If you feel you need more carbs for your sport or fitness goal, then do the NCD One Fruit Meal during the week, Mon-Sat, and FFSunday.™

Our target is 40 30 30, and we tweak the carbs down a bit for extra fat loss, or we adjust the carbs up some for additional energy for sports, or to gain size.™

HFFS is another option. Half-day of fruit meals, then switch to 40 30 30 for your last two meals of the day.™

The HFFS example on page 181 is a good fuel formula for the bodybuilder. Higher carbs 62%, less fat 14%, and good protein 24%, or about 60 15 25.™

60 15 25   can be tweaked to 56 13 31, more protein for your hard weightlifting workouts, just by adding in a second 250cal grilled chicken. Your body will be craving that extra chicken if you worked out hard and heavy.™

If you get the numbers right, you'll see results. If you fail to get this down, you'll be spinning your wheels, taking two-steps forward and two-steps back.™

It's no different than financial planning. You plug in the biweekly-contribution number, with the interest-rate number, and the time-frame number, hit calculate, and there's your nest egg, your result.

Mastering the numbers here, may help you to master the numbers elsewhere in your life. Numbers are Everywhere!™

The lowercarb tweak with the one peanuts substitution will make your end-of-the-day macros 31   42   27, if your daily is 2000. If your daily is 2500, then 33   40   27. Basically, flipping the carbs and fats from 40 30 30 to 30 40 30. This is moving you towards atkins, but not full atkins.™

This is a great way to cut carbs to 30%. And the 500 calories of peanuts will sustain you for 3 to 3½ hours, 4 hours maximum.™

Have beets, carrots, snap peas, cucumber, grapefruit, tomato, bell pepper, green beans, or any of the four "T" vegetables, broccoli, brussel sprouts, cauliflower, coleslaw, if you need something to carry you another 60 minutes until your next meal.™ (ABC NCD)

Won't you BE GLAD!! WHEN YOU ARRIVE AT YOUR IDEAL WEIGHT and you can eat your maintenance calories?

At your ideal weight, you have more freedom. When you're cutting calories, you have to pay more attention to your meal times.

NCD Blood-Glucose Range & Flags™
Target = 80 +/– 10   (or in Canada, 7 +/– 1)
Range = 70-90
Yellow Flag = 90s
Red Flag = 100s

Visualize that range diagram on page 184 when eating throughout your day. Stay between the lines, 70-90, or, 6-8 Feelin' Great!™

A one ProFat substitution with the 2000-calorie a day diet gives us macros of 31 39 30. Again, just flip the carb and fat percents.

If we have one ProFat and 4x 40 30 30 meals, 2500 calories per day, then our macros are 33 37 30. Basically, 30 40 30.

NCD Carb Tweaking™
Modifies the carbs from 30 40 50 55 60 70 80% carbs, with the fats concomitantly dropping from 40 30 25 15 15 0 0, while keeping the protein steady at 30 30 25 30 25 30 20.

40 30 30 is our Target – steady energy, and no food cravings.™

Fat cutting can be achieved in three ways. One, cut calories while keeping the macros the same, i.e., reduce 5x 40 30 30 to 4x 40 30 30. Or two, keep the calories the same but reduce the carbs, 5x 40 30 30 to 4x 40 30 30 plus 1x ProFat. Or, just add Cardio-Weights. And the fourth option, is to use any combination of the three.

The key thing is to, EAT WHAT YOU CRAVE AND GET IT OUT OF YOUR SYSTEM™

If you do that, you won't have any real desire for food after a while. You just eat because you know you have to.™

But that means getting your NUTRIENT STORES stocked up.™

Those shelves in your pantry need to be full of vitamins, minerals, omega-3, DHA EPA, phytonutrients, proteins, amino acids, and dozens of other nutrients that have yet to be named.™

Rather than eat for FEELing, eat for ENERGY. Sustained, steady, energy, glucose 80 +/- 10.™ Energy is what eating should give you. Because your meal is composed of calories, aka, Energy.™

Diet Isn't Half The Battle – It's The Whole Battle™

When treatments work, businesses lose customers. For some businesses this is fine, as there's another customer in the waiting room. For other business, especially businesses with a lot of overhead and expensive personnel, it is in their best interests to drag out your treatment, and this usually means poking at your problem from the front.™

Along with the word Discernment, the second word they don't want you to know or ask is, ROOT CAUSE. The medical system, as well as the alternative-health methods and systems, are both TREATMENT-based systems. Not ROOT CAUSE-based systems.

Jumper Publications go in from behind, fixing the foundation, the Root Causes of deterioration and aging.™

By Eliminating the Bad, and Adding In as Many of the Good as we can, the problem goes away as a Byproduct. The NCD Back Door.™

It's not important what your problem is, as the "fix" is the same for all problems. Eliminate the Bad. Add in the Good. Big problems are simply just small problems that have gotten worse over time. And those small problems may have morphed into something that appears completely unrelated to the big problems.™

When your Divine Intelligence runs short on supplies, it "robs-peter to pay-paul", and then your problem now shows up over there, as something else.™

The ABC Water and Number Crunch Diet address your foundation, and yes, fixing the foundation involves some work.™

Being fit and looking like you take care of yourself, i.e., your clothes fit well, earns you the respect of others.™

The respect of others makes you Untouchable.™

Your family, friends, and associates, will not give you a hard time.

You are Respected by all those you come in contact with.™

They take one look at you, and make an instant judgment based on how you look, and they treat you like a diplomat.™

You show to them that you take your appearance, health, body, skin, etc., seriously, so people take you seriously, they respect you.

You will find that life just goes your way a lot more often.™

When you look good, people leave you alone when it comes to cruelty, attitudes and remarks, in fact, they'll hold the door for you, move you to the front of the line, and give you discounts and freebies. They may actually "think" you're a celebrity.™

Life goes so much easier when you look good. That's just how people are. Our culture gives extra favor to those that look good.

When you take control of the numbers, you take control of how you look.™

When you take control of how you look, you take control of how you'll be treated.™

I know the person you want to be. The life you would rather have. It's real. You can have it. Do your part, and it's yours.

So by going in through the backdoor, by fixing your nutrition, your calorie intake, and your poor-food choices, the fat comes off.

When the fat comes off, your hormones fall into place as a byproduct.™ Hormonal Regulation just happens. You wake up one morning and it occurs to you, it's gone, that problem's gone.™

By drinking alkaline water you perform a full body detox, the fat falls off and you have less fatigue so your energy goes up so you need less calories and the fat falls off some more. It's a vicious cycle. But a good vicious cycle.™

NCD Skillet Chicken & Carrot Cake™

NCD Skillet Chicken & Buttered Popcorn™

This is the only diet that gives you complete nutrition, with maximum freedom, combined with total control.™

It's really the "All Your Dreams Come True Control Freak" diet.™

With a side of entertainment!

Oh, and the Chocolate Mayonnaise Cake! That one is pure heaven. And it's so simple to make. Easy to make, but not easy to bake, because if you undercook it it turns into chocolate mayonnaise fudge cake! And we can't have that. Actually, we can!

That recipe will have to wait until the next volume of TCY. But you can relax, knowing that the dessert is not going to make you gain weight because it's the carbfat portion of the meal. Those yummy melt-in-your-mouth numbers are built into the meal as your 200 calories of carbs and 150 calories of fat. You just have to have a protein. And your vegetable!

God Bless You!

You! are! a true winner! Go out there and win some more, and through word-of-mouth, who knows how many lives can be impacted. Self-Health Options need their place at the "table". Otherwise, we're all gonna die!, if traditional ways of doing things stay as they are. If this material has helped you, tell a friend.

Chapter Endnote
Okay, you're hungry again and you're still away from home, what now? Jack-In-The-Box. Order two Chicken Fajita Pita, just the pitas/sandwiches, not the combo!   E=568 F=166 CHO=237 Na=2211mg!!! Prot=172,   41.5   28.4   30.1, or with the fiber subtracted, about 40 30 30. Chase this with a glass of water later. $10.51, they're charging you for the extra salt!

Leave a Review

Without giving away the contents, "spoilers", recommend this publication and leave a review so that someone else might benefit from it too. Thank you.

www.amazon.com   Search: 12 Changes A Year

Subscribe to my YouTube Channel
www.youtube.com   Search: Number Crunch Diet

Be sure to send me an email so I can periodically keep in touch with updates and new Selfcare Strategies – and discount offers on new items (yes, more than books!) (a simple and effective weight-loss device) (a weightlifting "device" that I use EVERY time I work out) and don't forget – TCY Volume 2!

abcwaterandthenumbercrunchdiet@mail.com
Privacy – your email address will not be used for anything other than by Jumper Publications and Media.

I almost forgot! (again, not really) to tell you!

If you liked this shake recipe be sure to check out

TCY
12 Changes a Year
Vol 2

for the NCD ORANGE SHAKE!
It makes 9, and I often repeat the recipe midweek.
And whey protein – but not from powder.
And not from cottage cheese either!

BUY THE BOOK!!
IT'S GOOD STUFF!

Saliva vs Urine pH

Top Ten Reasons Why Saliva pH Is Worthless When Compared To Urine pH For Acid-Base Analysis

#10 Small Volume – small tiny volume samples don't represent the whole

#9 Difficult to Obtain – the procedure is to bring up saliva and swallow, 2x, then use the third one for the test, too hard to obtain

#8 Poor Reproducibility – when you retest your saliva sample, you will likely get a slightly different color (reading)

#7 Poor Accuracy – if you collect a second sample, it will likely give you a different reading than the first

#6 Bacterial Contamination – bacteria from your mouth will interfere with the test

#5 Food Contamination – food from your mouth will interfere with the test

#4 Spoon Contamination – the surface of the spoon that you collect it on is going to affect your small sample

#3 Viscosity – saliva is too thick and results in faded or dual colors of the test pad (or paper)

#2 Difficulty Reading – the color doesn't "lock in" so you can take a reading, it tends to change shades through a range

#1 Your Salivary Glands have ZERO to do with Acid-Base regulation. Try Kidneys.

Your kidneys are running your body's alkaline status.

And your alkaline status is the secret they don't want you to know.

JPM Oral Hygiene Protocol

This publication is the introduction to JPM. If you paid $2.99 for the kindle version or $4.99 for the paperback version, then you basically paid for the two protocols, the 20% vodka mouthwash, and the Secret Weapon, H_2O_2 gum-line cleaner. You will notice advertising for the other publications. Don't be upset. You got your $3-5 worth. The same cost as for a venti mocha latte, that's long since gone. The information in this publication will be with you for you to use for the rest of your life, every day.

So, why not take the ABC NCD Quiz!

The first half of the book is all about alkalinity. The secret aspect to your health no one, but a few, will talk about. However, no one covers the subject better and more comprehensively than in ABC Water™. The second half is the Number Crunch Diet™. No recipes, but lots of good sound information on diet. You will learn a lot, as no one discusses it the way I do. I brag a bit about the book, because it's really a great book. It's a compilation of nearly 100 books that I've read. But more of a Synergy, a new approach.

The recipes can be found in *12 Changes A Year* and you can see a sample on www.abcwaterandthenumbercrunchdiet.com

The title *Nontoxic Teeth Whitening and Dental Hygiene System* begins with the two chapters you just read, but includes a one-of-a-kind food-grade teeth whitening system, if you feel you need more whitening. It also includes a commentary on fluoride. Wouldn't you like to know if fluoride's something you should be doing, or something you shouldn't be doing?

So put your thinking cap on and let's start the Quiz!

It's good for you!

Pick the correct answers – There may be more than one

1. A urine pH of 5 is telling you
   a. about your blood pressure
   b. that you're tired
   c. about your alkaline reserves
   d. to see a doctor
   e. that you're healthy and fine

2. Urine pH testing is routinely performed by licensed
   a. social workers
   b. clinical laboratory scientists
   c. respiratory therapists
   d. fitness advisors
   e. nurses and doctors

3. The cost of one month of urine pH testing is _____ the cost of open heart surgery (CABG).
   a. 1/10
   b. 1/100
   c. 1/1000
   d. 1/10,000
   e. 1/100,000

4. The opposite of metabolic acid is dietary
   a. phosphates – found in meats and cola drinks
   b. bicarbonate – found in packaged foods
   c. caffeine – found in green tea
   d. bicarbonate – found in fruits and vegetables
   e. bicarbonate – found in oils and fats

5. Information can be of which types
   a. true
   b. incomplete

c. false
d. clouded
e. secret

6. "Natural Flavor" on a food label is
   a. natural flavor extracts from plants and fruit
   b. glutamates, MSG, altered salts
   c. chemicals that make you addicted to the product
   d. generally safe and good for me
   e. not something I need to worry about

7. During World War II, the people who failed to act early
   a. suffered
   b. died
   c. lost everything
   d. became victims
   e. made it through unscathed

8. Compensating means
   a. saving for retirement
   b. eating foods that lift your mood
   c. doing something to mask something
   d. brushing it out of your thoughts
   e. pleasing others and being a do-gooder
   f. all of the above

9. The reason(s) people are fat
   a. they're born that way
   b. they don't make their own meals
   c. hereditary – handed down from your parents
   d. my body just won't lose fat
   e. they don't see the numbers in what they're eating

10. The "Cheat Day" is
    a. a great way to get food cravings satisfied
    b. required to reset my fat-burning hormones
    c. a 2-8 step backwards day
    d. works well for most people long term
    e. is a popular "trick" that you should buy into

ANSWERS

1. A urine pH of 5 is telling you
    a. about your blood pressure – No, but there is a relationship
       (see Chapter 24)
    b. that you're tired – No, but there is a relationship (see Chapter
       20)
    c. about your alkaline reserves – YES! Get to know your
       alkaline status by reading this book.
    d. to see a doctor – No, but it can lead to that.
    e. that you're healthy and fine – One number tells you little, 35
       numbers a week tells you a lot. Get to know your urine pH.

2. Urine pH testing is routinely performed by licensed
    a. social workers – no
    b. clinical laboratory scientists – Yes, 99% of all urine testing is
       done by a CLS.
    c. respiratory therapists – no
    d. fitness advisors – no
    e. nurses and doctors – Doctors do perform urine tests in their
       offices, but they are not looking at urine pH with much depth.

3. The cost of one month of urine pH testing is _____ the cost of
   open heart surgery (CABG)(a bypass, "cabbage").
    a. 1/10 – no
    b. 1/100 – no
    c. 1/1000 – no
    d. 1/10,000 – Yes. You can test all of your urinations for about

$1 a month (see Chapter 11). A cabbage would run you at least $10,000.

e. 1/100,000 – no. But I believe the potential to save yourself $100,000 in medical treatments is very possible.

4. The opposite of metabolic acid is dietary
   a. phosphates – no, phosphates contribute to acidity
   b. bicarbonate – no, bicarbonate yes, but not from packaged foods
   c. caffeine – no, caffeine is a drug, most drugs are acidic
   d. bicarbonate found in fruits and vegetables – Yes!
   e. bicarbonate found in oils and fats – no, oils and fats are not sources of bicarbonate

5. Information can be of which types
   a. true – Yes, this is a bit what your life is all about. Finding the truth about things.
   b. incomplete – aka, partial truths or half truths, aka, "spin". Do you find your head spinning when you go for fancy medical treatments?
   c. false – lies, yes lies. Don't call them untruths. Lies are Lies. When people lie it's your job to call them on it. Otherwise, "ya got no backbone".
   d. clouded – blurry, muddied, confusion. I could write "scientifically" but I would just make you confused and half lost. How does that help you.
   e. secret – Now we're talking. When they say "buy this stock" you've got to be a moron to buy it. The payoffs and the winners are kept secret, shared through word of mouth.

6. "Natural Flavor" on a food label is
   a. natural flavor extracts from plants and fruit – Well, they would like you to think that, but that's far from reality.
   b. glutamates, MSG, altered salts – Yes, often this is the case.
   c. chemicals that make you addicted to the product – Yes

Absolutely
d. generally safe and good for me – don't buy that line
e. not something I need to worry about – you make your own choices in life

7. During World War II, the people that failed to act early
Referring to this is grim and bleak. But there are people suffering and dying every day because they failed to act early. You could say that WWII is still happening all around us in the United States of America today. My book can help you not to fall victim to this death and suffering. So that you make it through your life, unscathed.

8. Compensating means
   a. saving for retirement – no, but I have seen people who are just a little too attached to their portfolios, compensating?
   b. eating foods that lift your mood – no, but food is commonly used to compensate
   c. doing something to mask something – Ah-Ha, Yes.
   d. brushing it out of your thoughts – no. It's okay and healthy to let go of thoughts, just be sure you're not avoiding your issues.
   e. people pleasing – reward seekers may be compensating
   f. all of the above – no, just C. Go back and read C again.

9. The reason(s) people are fat
   a. they're born that way – don't give me that
   b. they don't make their own meals – Bingo! This is key.
   c. heredity – your fat jeans are because of your fat genes – no I don't think so
   d. my body just won't lose fat – I hear you. There is not a lot of good help out there. Luckily, you've found the right place.
   e. they don't see the numbers in what they're eating – Yes. And person D above just needs to look at food mathematically (and read the book).

10. The "Cheat Day" is
   a. a great way to get food cravings satisfied – Wrong. I'm a testimony of getting rid of food cravings. See Chapter 38, 39, 40, 41.
   b. required to reset my fat-burning hormones – Wrong. If you get your macros right, your hormones will cooperate just fine.
   c. a 2-8 step backwards day – On page 84 of *The Four Hour Body* the person states that he gains 4.4 lbs on his cheat day. Then he loses it. Can you say "moody"?
   d. works well for most people long term – After reading dozens of diet books, I could not find one that worked long term, so I made my own. It's called the Number Crunch Diet.
   e. a popular "trick" that you should buy into – The Number Crunch Diet isn't about cheating. Although it's full of useful "tricks" that I came up with and use daily.

You'll be miles ahead of the average person after a while.

If you've read ABC NCD & TCY, then you already are!

Now add *The 5 Points of Posture* for the polished touch!